The Labour Ward Handbook

This succinct manual provides detailed clinical practice guidelines for the care of women in labour; it is designed to be a ready guide for use in the delivery suite by the busy clinician. The third edition has been updated to include new developments in clinical practice and governance and new guidelines. So far as is possible, the differences in care scenarios internationally have been addressed to provide a reliable guide to safe delivery.

Prof Edozien was a Consultant in Obstetrics and Gynaecology at St Mary's Hospital, Manchester, UK, and is currently Professor and Director of the Institute of Advanced Clinical Sciences Education, University of Medical Sciences, Ondo City, Nigeria.

The Labour Ward Handbook
Third Edition

Leroy C Edozien
LLB MBBS BSc MSc MPhil PhD MRCPI FRCOG FWACS
Former Consultant in Obstetrics and Gynaecology,
St Mary's Hospital, Manchester, UK
Professor & Director, Institute of Advanced Clinical Sciences Education,
University of Medical Sciences, Ondo City, Nigeria

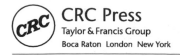
CRC Press
Taylor & Francis Group
Boca Raton London New York

CRC Press is an imprint of the
Taylor & Francis Group, an **informa** business

Cover Image © Shutterstock images

Third edition published 2024
by CRC Press
6000 Broken Sound Parkway NW, Suite 300, Boca Raton, FL 33487–2742

and by CRC Press
4 Park Square, Milton Park, Abingdon, Oxon, OX14 4RN

CRC Press is an imprint of Taylor & Francis Group, LLC

© 2024 Taylor & Francis Group, LLC

Second edition published by Hodder Arnold, 2011

This book contains information obtained from authentic and highly regarded sources. While all reasonable efforts have been made to publish reliable data and information, neither the author nor the publisher can accept any legal responsibility or liability for any errors or omissions that may be made. The publishers wish to make clear that any views or opinions expressed in this book by individual editors, authors or contributors are personal to them and do not necessarily reflect the views/opinions of the publishers. The information or guidance contained in this book is intended for use by medical, scientific or healthcare professionals and is provided strictly as a supplement to the medical or other professional's own judgement, their knowledge of the patient's medical history, relevant manufacturer's instructions and the appropriate best practice guidelines. Because of the rapid advances in medical science, any information or advice on dosages, procedures or diagnoses should be independently verified. The reader is strongly urged to consult the relevant national drug formulary and the drug companies' and device or material manufacturers' printed instructions, and their websites, before administering or utilizing any of the drugs, devices or materials mentioned in this book. This book does not indicate whether a particular treatment is appropriate or suitable for a particular individual. Ultimately it is the sole responsibility of the medical professional to make his or her own professional judgements, so as to advise and treat patients appropriately. The authors and publishers have also attempted to trace the copyright holders of all material reproduced in this publication and apologize to copyright holders if permission to publish in this form has not been obtained. If any copyright material has not been acknowledged please write and let us know so we may rectify in any future reprint.

Library of Congress Cataloging-in-Publication Data
Names: Edozien, Leroy C., author.
Title: The labour ward handbook / Leroy C Edozien.
Description: Third edition. | Boca Raton, FL : CRC Press, 2023. | Includes bibliographical references and index.
Identifiers: LCCN 2023000361 (print) | LCCN 2023000362 (ebook) | ISBN 9781138296633 (paperback) |
    ISBN 9781138296640 (hardback) | ISBN 9781315099897 (ebook)
Subjects: MESH: Labor, Obstetric | Handbook
Classification: LCC RG525 (print) | LCC RG525 (ebook) | NLM WQ 39 | DDC 618.2—dc23/eng/20230429
LC record available at https://lccn.loc.gov/2023000361
LC ebook record available at https://lccn.loc.gov/2023000362

ISBN: 978-1-138-29664-0 (hbk)
ISBN: 978-1-138-29663-3 (pbk)
ISBN: 978-1-315-09989-7 (ebk)

DOI: 10.1201/9781315099897

For
Orange Mummy

Contents

Preface   xxi
Acknowledgements   xxii
About the Author   xxiii
Abbreviations   xxiv
Glossary   xxvi
Bleep/crash calls   xxvii

PART I   Approach to care   **1**

1 The biopsychosocial approach to care of the woman in labour   **3**
   1.1   Assessing women's satisfaction with intrapartum care   5

2 Communication between care providers   **6**
   2.1   Early identification and communication of risk   6
   2.2   Handover   7
   2.3   Communication with anaesthetists   7

3 Documentation   **9**

4 Admission to, and discharge home from, the delivery suite   **10**
   4.1   Admission   10
   4.2   Discharge   10

5 Learning from clinical incidents   **11**
   5.1   What is a clinical incident?   11
   5.2   Why do we need clinical incident analysis?   12
   5.3   Reporting clinical incidents   12
   5.4   Learning from clinical incidents   12
   5.5   Confidentiality   13

6 Transfer of care between professionals   **14**
   6.1   Background   14
   6.2   Handover by clinical staff   14
   6.3   Transfer of emergencies from primary care   14
   6.4   Transfer between hospitals with the fetus in utero   15
   6.5   Transfer of care between consultants   15
   6.6   Transfer back to the community or GP care   15
   6.7   Transfer to ICU and HDU   16
   6.8   Who is in charge while the woman is in ICU or HDU?   16
   6.9   Return to delivery suite from ICU   16

7 Reviewing what happened   **17**

Further reading for Part I   **18**

PART II   Normal and Low-Risk Labour   **19**

8 Vaginal examination   **21**
   8.1   Before vaginal examination   21
   8.2   During vaginal examination   21
   8.3   Details to be recorded   21

9 Intravenous cannulation   **22**

10 Management of normal labour   **23**
   10.1   Criteria for normal labour   23

11 Prelabour rupture of membranes at term (37–42 weeks)   **24**
   11.1   Further management   25
   11.2   Expectant management   25
   11.3   Active management   26

12 Management of the first stage of labour   **27**
   12.1   Diagnosis   27
   12.2   Monitoring progress of labour   27
   12.3   Birth plans   28
   12.4   Support person   28
   12.5   Positioning   28
   12.6   Nutrition   28
   12.7   Antacids (including H2-receptor antagonists)   28
   12.8   Pain relief   29
   12.9   Entonox (50% O_2 and 50% N_2O)   29
   12.10 Opioids (pethidine, diamorphine or other)   29
   12.11 Epidural analgesia   30
   12.12 Bladder care   30

13 Fetal monitoring   **31**
   13.1   Intermittent auscultation   31
   13.2   Electronic fetal monitoring   31
   13.3   Suspicious or abnormal trace   32
   13.4   Classification of cardiotocograph (Table 13.1)   32
   13.5   Management of suspicious or pathological cardiotocograph   32
   13.6   Management of fetal tachycardia   34
   13.7   Note   34
   13.8   Management of fetal bradycardia   34
   13.9   Schedule   35
   13.10 Reduced variability (2–5 beats/min)   35
   13.11 Late deceleration   35

14 Fetal scalp blood sampling   **37**
    14.1   Contraindications to FBS   37
    14.2   Interpretation of pH result   37
    14.3   Scalp blood lactate   38
    14.4   Documentation   38
    14.5   FBS at full cervical dilatation   38

15 Augmentation of labour   **39**
    15.1   Artificial rupture of fetal membranes (ARM)   39
    15.2   Augmentation with Syntocinon   40
    15.3   Syntocinon infusion   40
    15.4   Second stage of labour   41
    15.5   Uterine hyperstimulation   41
    15.6   Management   41

16 Cord-blood sampling   **42**

17 Epidural analgesia in labour   **43**
    17.1   Indications for epidural analgesia   43
    17.2   Contraindications to epidural analgesia   43
    17.3   Coagulopathy   44
    17.4   Therapeutic/prophylactic anticoagulation   44
    17.5   Setting up   44
    17.6   Procedure   45
    17.7   Method of administration   45
    17.8   Epidural infusion   45
    17.9   Epidural top-up   46
    17.10 Protocol for top-ups   46
    17.11 General care of the woman with an epidural   47
    17.12 In the second stage of labour   48
    17.13 Complications of epidural analgesia   48
    17.14 Dural tap   48
    17.15 Local anaesthetic toxicity (IV injection)   49
    17.16 Total spinal   49
    17.17 Dense motor block   49
    17.18 Bladder distension   50
    17.19 Discontinuation of epidural   50

18 Management of the second stage of labour   **51**
    18.1   Duration   51
    18.2   Passive phase   51
    18.3   Active phase   52
    18.4   Immediate versus delayed pushing   52
    18.5   Delayed second stage   52
    18.6   Management of delayed second stage   53
    18.7   Calling the paediatrician   53

19 Criteria for paediatric attendance at delivery   **54**

20 Management of the third stage of labour   **55**
  20.1 Active management   55
  20.2 If the placenta is not delivered within 30 minutes, refer to the obstetrician 56
  20.3 Physiological management   56

21 Immediate postpartum care   **57**
  21.1 Care of the mother   57
  21.2 Bladder care   57
  21.3 Care of the baby   58
  21.4 The placenta   58
  21.5 Documentation   58

22 Care of the newborn   **59**
  22.1 Skin-to-skin contact   59
  22.2 Prevention of hypothermia   59
  22.3 Vitamin K   60
  22.4 Identification of the baby   60
  22.5 Breastfeeding   61
  22.6 Management of hypoglycaemia   61
  22.7 Preventive care   61

23 Meconium-stained amniotic fluid   **62**
  23.1 Risk to baby   62
  23.2 Note   62
  23.3 Meconium-stained fluid in labour   62
  23.4 Meconium-stained fluid at vaginal delivery   62
  23.5 Meconium-stained fluid at caesarean section   63

24 Neonatal resuscitation   **64**
  24.1 Principles   64
  24.2 Avoid thermal stress   64
  24.3 Airway   65
  24.4 Evaluation   65
  24.5 Breathing   65
  24.6 Chest compression   67
  24.7 Drugs used in neonatal resuscitation   67
  24.8 Volume replacement   68

25 Babies born before arrival at hospital   **69**
  25.1 Mother   69
  25.2 Baby   69

26 Episiotomy   **70**

27 The woman with a history of childhood sexual abuse   **71**
  27.1 General measures   71
  27.2 Communication   71
  27.3 Physical examination and procedures   71
  27.4 Flashbacks   72

28 Use of birthing pool   **73**
   28.1 Inclusion criteria   73
   28.2 Exclusion criteria   73
   28.3 Conduct of labour   74
   28.4 Support in labour   74
   28.5 Indications for asking the woman to leave the pool   74
   28.6 Delivery   75
   28.7 General   75

   Further reading for Part II   **76**

PART III Abnormal and high-risk labour   **81**

SECTION 1 Powers, passenger, passage   *83*

29 Caesarean section   **85**
   29.1 Preparations   85
   29.2 Medication to reduce the risk of aspiration syndrome   85
   29.3 Classification of urgency of CS   86
   29.4 Elective CS   86
   29.5 Workplace noise   87
   29.6 Emergency CS   87
   29.7 Surgical procedure   87
   29.8 Prophylactic antibiotics   88
   29.9 High-risk cases   88
   29.10 Delayed elective CS   88
   29.11 Postoperative care   88
   29.12 Thromboprophylaxis   89

30 Recovery of obstetric patients   **90**

31 High-dependency care   **92**
   31.1 Early warning score   92

32 Failed intubation drill   **94**

33 Instrumental delivery   **95**
   33.1 Non-operative interventions which reduce instrumental delivery rates   95
   33.2 Avoiding harm   95
   33.3 Indications for instrumental delivery   95
   33.4 Conditions to be fulfilled before instrumental delivery   96
   33.5 Classification of instrumental vaginal delivery   96
   33.6 Communication   96
   33.7 Choice of instrument   97
   33.8 Pre-application assessment: abdominal and vaginal examination   97
   33.9 Vacuum-assisted delivery   99
   33.10 Procedure   99
   33.11 Contraindications to vacuum-assisted delivery   100
   33.12 Forceps delivery   100

33.13 Checking for proper application of the forceps   101
33.14 Kjelland forceps   101
33.15 Trial of instrumental delivery   101
33.16 The principle of abandonment   102
33.17 Post-delivery   102
33.18 Documentation   103
33.19 Errors in instrumental vaginal delivery   103

34 Trial of vaginal delivery after a previous caesarean section   106
34.1   Contraindications   106
34.2   Action plan for trial of vaginal delivery   106
34.3   Use of Syntocinon   107
34.4   Signs of scar rupture or imminent rupture   107
34.5   Post-delivery   107

35 Induction of labour   108
35.1   Methods   108
35.2   Artificial rupture of fetal membranes   109
35.3   Prostaglandin induction of labour   111
35.4   Monitoring following insertion of prostaglandin   112
35.5   Precautions   112
35.6   Hyperstimulation   112
35.7   Syntocinon infusion   112
35.8   Uterine hyperstimulation   113

36 Antenatal corticosteroid therapy   114
36.1   Indications   114
36.2   Dose   114
36.3   Contraindications   114
36.4   Beta-sympathomimetics   115
36.5   Repeated doses   115

37 Preterm prelabour rupture of membranes   116
37.1   Action plan   116
37.2   Conservative management   117
37.3   Mode of delivery, in the absence of other complications 117
37.4   Induction of labour   117
37.5   Labour   117

38 Preterm uterine contractions   118
38.1   Diagnosis   118
38.2   Action plan   118
38.3   Fetal fibronectin test   119
38.4   Management of established preterm labour (when it is too late to
       suppress labour)   119
38.5   Suppression of labour   120
38.6   Contraindications to suppression of labour   120
38.7   Nifedipine   121
38.8   Indomethacin (prostaglandins synthetase inhibitor)   122
38.9   Atosiban   122

38.10   Magnesium sulphate for neuroprotection   123
38.11   Monitoring   123

39   Deliveries at the lower margin of viability   **124**
39.1   Pregnancy under 22 weeks   124
39.2   Pregnancy over 22 weeks   124
39.3   Post-delivery care if the baby does not survive   125
39.4   Support group   125

40   Multiple pregnancy   **126**
40.1   First stage of labour   126
40.2   Second stage of labour   127
40.3   Delivery of the second twin   127
40.4   Third stage of labour   129
40.5   Indications for CS for second twin   129

41   Abnormal lie in labour   **130**
41.1   Intact membranes   130
41.2   Ruptured membranes   130
41.3   Caesarean section   130
41.4   Difficult cases   131
41.5   Uterodistension   131

42   Occipito-posterior position   **132**
42.1   Persistent occipito-posterior position   132

43   Malpresentation   **133**
43.1   Brow presentation   133
43.2   Face presentation   133
43.3   Compound presentation   134

44   Breech presentation   **135**
44.1   Undiagnosed breech in labour   135
44.2   Preterm breech in labour   135
44.3   Breech vaginal delivery   136
44.4   Caesarean section for breech presentation (elective or emergency)   137

45   External cephalic version   **138**
45.1   Risks of ECV   138
45.2   Contraindications to ECV   138
45.3   Cautions   138
45.4   Action plan   139

46   The woman with genital cutting   **140**
46.1   WHO classification of female genital cutting   140
46.2   Action plan   140
46.3   Female Genital Mutilation Act 2003   141

47   The obese woman in labour   **142**
47.1   WHO classification of BMI   142
47.2   Woman who had bariatric surgery   143

48 Perineal tear   **144**
   48.1   Classification of perineal tears   144
   48.2   First- and second-degree tears: episiotomy   144
   48.3   Third- and fourth-degree tears   145

SECTION 2   *Medical conditions*   **147**

49 Heart disease in labour   **149**
   49.1   Principles of management   149
   49.2   Action plan   150

50 Peripartum cardiomyopathy   **152**
   50.1   Diagnosis   152
   50.2   Risk factors   152
   50.3   Symptoms and signs   152
   50.4   Action plan   153

51 Pre-eclampsia   **154**
   51.1   Classification   154
   51.2   Action plan   155
   51.3   Measurement of blood pressure   155
   51.4   Severe pre-eclampsia   156
   51.5   Delivery   157
   51.6   Watch for PPH   157
   51.7   Post-delivery   157
   51.8   Antihypertensive therapy in pre-eclampsia   157
   51.9   Labetalol   158
  51.10   Hydralazine   158
  51.11   Nifedipine   159
  51.12   Anticonvulsant prophylaxis in pre-eclampsia   159
  51.13   Magnesium sulphate blood levels   160
  51.14   Management of magnesium toxicity   160
  51.15   Postpartum   160
  51.16   Post-delivery ward round (days 0–3)   161
  51.17   Fluid management in pre-eclampsia   161
  51.18   Management of oliguria (<80 mL in 4 hours)   163
  51.19   Blood transfusion   163

52 Eclampsia   **164**
   52.1   Action plan   164
   52.2   Anticonvulsant treatment (magnesium sulphate)   164
   52.3   Magnesium sulphate blood levels   165
   52.4   Persistent seizures   165
   52.5   Controlling blood pressure   166
   52.6   General management   166

53 Diabetes mellitus   **167**
   53.1   Recommended timing of delivery   167
   53.2   Induction of labour by artificial rupture of fetal membranes   167

53.3   Induction of labour with prostaglandin   167
53.4   Elective caesarean section   168
53.5   First stage of labour   168
53.6   Gestational diabetes, diet-controlled   169
53.7   Preterm labour   170
53.8   After delivery   170
53.9   Care of the neonate   170
53.10 Maternal hypoglycaemic shock   171
53.11 Diabetic ketoacidosis   171
53.12 Presentation   171

54 Asthma (acute exacerbation in labour)   **173**
54.1   Drugs that can cause or aggravate bronchospasm   173
54.2   Action points   173
54.3   After delivery   174

55 Epilepsy   **175**
55.1   Management in labour   175
55.2   Indications for caesarean section   175
55.3   Management of fits in labour   175
55.4   After seizure   176
55.5   After delivery   176

56 Systemic lupus erythematosus   **178**
56.1   Principles   178
56.2   Action plan   178
56.3   Neonatal lupus   179

57 Connective tissue disorders   **180**
57.1   Rheumatoid arthritis   180
57.2   Marfan syndrome   180
57.3   Ehlers–Danlos syndrome   181

SECTION 3   Haemorrhage and haematological disorders   **183**

58 The rhesus-negative woman   **185**
58.1   Sensitizing events   185
58.2   At delivery   185
58.3   Transfusions   186

59 Thromboembolism prophylaxis   **187**
59.1   Thromboprophylaxis for caesarean section   187
59.2   Low risk   187
59.3   Moderate risk   188
59.4   High risk   188
59.5   Thromboprophylaxis in vaginal deliveries   189
59.6   Low risk   189
59.7   Moderate risk   189
59.8   High risk   190

59.9   Relative and absolute contraindications to the use of dalteparin   190
59.10   The use of unfractionated heparin (UFH)   190
59.11   Regional analgesia   191
59.12   Regional analgesia and dalteparin   191

60 Acute venous thromboembolism and pulmonary embolism   **192**
60.1   Risk factors   192
60.2   Clinical features   192
60.3   Initial investigations   193
60.4   Suspected DVT   193
60.5   Suspected PE   193
60.6   Anticoagulant therapy for DVT and PE   194
60.7   Duration of treatment   196
60.8   Labour and delivery   196
60.9   High risk woman on *therapeutic* LMWH   197
60.10   Woman on high dose *prophylaxis*, twice-a-day regimen   197
60.11   Induction of labour   197
60.12   Elective caesarean section   197
60.13   Third stage of labour   198
60.14   Epidural or spinal anaesthesia   198
60.15   Postpartum anticoagulation   198

61 Major haemoglobinopathy   **199**
61.1   Principles of management in labour   199
61.2   Action plan   199
61.3   Sickle cell crisis   200
61.4   Action plan   200

62 Inherited coagulation disorders: Haemophilia and von Willebrand disease   **202**
62.1   Haemophilia   202
62.2   Von Willebrand disease   203
62.3   Action plan   203
62.4   The neonate   204

63 Immune thrombocytopenic purpura   **205**
63.1   Differential diagnoses of thrombocytopenia in pregnancy   205
63.2   Action plan   205
63.3   Mode of delivery   206
63.4   The neonate   206
63.5   Postnatal care   206

64 Thrombophilia   **207**
64.1   Management in labour   207
64.2   Epidural analgesia   207
64.3   Postpartum   208

65 Gestational thrombocytopenia   **209**

66 Antepartum haemorrhage   **210**
66.1   RCOG classification of APH   210
66.2   Differential diagnoses   210

66.3   Placental abruption   210
66.4   Assessment   211
66.5   Minor APH (minimal loss, <50 mL on admission)   211
66.6   Major APH (significant bleeding, 50–1000 mL but not in shock)   211
66.7   Massive APH (estimated loss >1000 mL and/or signs of clinical shock)   211
66.8   Delivery   213

67   Major placenta praevia   **214**
67.1   Action plan   214
67.2   Cell salvage   215

68   Placenta accreta spectrum   **216**
68.1   Investigation   216
68.2   Delivery   216

69   Retained placenta   **218**
69.1   Action plan   218

70   Postpartum haemorrhage   **219**
70.1   Action plan   219
70.2   Retained placenta   220
70.3   Uterine atony   220
70.4   Genital tract trauma or undiagnosed bleeding   221
70.5   Coagulopathy   221
70.6   Transfusion of blood products   221
70.7   Compression suture   222
70.8   Where could things go wrong?   223
70.9   Documentation   223

71   Disseminated intravascular coagulopathy   **225**
71.1   Investigations   225
71.2   Treatment   225

72   Delivery of the woman at known risk of haemorrhage   **226**
72.1   If surgery is indicated   226

73   Standards for administering blood transfusion   **228**
73.1   Background   228
73.2   Obtaining consent   229
73.3   Collecting a specimen for group-and-save/cross-match   229
73.4   Checking procedure for blood transfusion   229
73.5   Documentation   230

74   Management of the woman who declines blood transfusion   **231**
74.1   Antenatal care   231
74.2   Labour   232
74.3   Management of haemorrhage   232
74.4   Communication   232
74.5   Drugs and infusions   233
74.6   Hysterectomy   233
74.7   Management of staff   233

SECTION 4   *Infection*   **235**

75 Prophylactic antibiotics   **237**
   75.1 Caesarean section   237
   75.2 Cardiac disease (see Chapter 49)   237
   75.3 Group B streptococci (GBS)   238
   75.4 Prolonged rupture of fetal membranes   238

76 Intrapartum sepsis   **239**
   76.1 Principles   239
   76.2 Action plan   239

77 Hepatitis B and C   **241**
   77.1 Action plan   241
   77.2 Immunization   241
   77.3 Breastfeeding   242

78 Intrapartum antibiotic prophylaxis for Group B streptococci   **243**
   78.1 Principles   243
   78.2 Risk factors   243
   78.3 Indications for intrapartum GBS prophylaxis   243
   78.4 Intrapartum GBS prophylaxis not indicated   244
   78.5 Action plan   244
   78.6 Neonate   244
   78.7 Useful contact for patients   246
   78.8 Helpline 0330 120 0796 (UK)   246

79 Genital herpes   **247**

80 Human immunodeficiency virus   **249**
   80.1 Mode of delivery   249
   80.2 Management of vaginal delivery   250
   80.3 Other measures to reduce the risk of vertical transmission   250
   80.4 After delivery   250
   80.5 Breastfeeding   251
   80.6 Preparation for caesarean section   251
   80.7 Prelabour rupture of membranes at term (PROM)   251
   80.8 Preterm prelabour rupture of membranes   251
   80.9 Cord blood   251
  80.10 Care of the baby   252
  80.11 Infection control   252

81 The woman with COVID-19   **253**
   81.1 Action plan   253
   81.2 Clinical care   253

SECTION 5 Other obstetric emergencies 255

82 Paravaginal haematoma and cervical tear 257
82.1 Paravaginal haematoma 257
82.2 Cervical tear 258

83 Rupture of the uterus 259
83.1 Action plan 259
83.2 Preventive care 259

84 Shoulder dystocia 261
84.1 Risk factors 261
84.2 Risks to mother and baby 261
84.3 When shoulder dystocia is anticipated 261
84.4 Turtle sign 262
84.5 Action plan: 'HELPERR' 262
84.6 After delivery 263
84.7 Documentation 263

85 Cord prolapse 264
85.1 Risk factors 264
85.2 Action plan 264

86 Anaphylaxis 266
86.1 Presentation 266
86.2 World Allergy Organization criteria for diagnosis of anaphylaxis 266
86.3 Action plan 267

87 Inverted uterus 268
87.1 Action plan 268
87.2 Reduction of the inversion 268
87.3 Hydrostatic reduction 269

88 Amniotic fluid embolism 270
88.1 Differential diagnoses 270
88.2 Management 270

89 Sudden maternal collapse 272
89.1 Possible causes 272
89.2 Management 272
89.3 Investigations 273

90 Latex allergy 274
90.1 Risk factors 274
90.2 Care of the woman allergic to latex 274
90.3 Operating theatre (elective or emergency procedure) 275

SECTION 6   Stillbirths and congenital abnormalities   277

91 Checklist for fetal loss at 13–23 weeks   **279**
   91.1   Parents   279
   91.2   Communication   279
   91.3   Forms/administration   • 279

92 Intrauterine fetal demise   **280**
   92.1   Principles   280
   92.2   Diagnosis (if not made before admission)   280
   92.3   Action plan   281
   92.4   Investigations   281
   92.5   Induction of labour   282
   92.6   Support group   283

93 Mid-trimester termination of pregnancy for fetal abnormality   **284**
   93.1   Investigations   284
   93.2   Prenatal diagnosis of chromosomal abnormality   284
   93.3   Ultrasound scan diagnosis of structural abnormality or external appearance
       suggestive of aneuploidy   284
   93.4   Scan diagnosis of neural tube defect, with no other malformation or recurrences
       in family   285
   93.5   Genetic examination of fetuses and samples   285
   93.6   Induction of labour   285
   93.7   Contraindications   286
   93.8   Caution   286

Further reading for Part III   **287**

Appendix   298
Index   301

Preface

In high pressure situations such as the delivery suite, clinical practice guidelines can be invaluable. Unfortunately, many guidelines are written in the form of a textbook of theory and practice, not in a style that facilitates speedy reference. What busy staff *on the shop floor* need in the delivery suite is not a tome that describes underlying theories and research findings, but a handbook that succinctly spells out what should be done and when. *The Labour Ward Handbook* sets out to meet this need. The layout is reader-friendly, with less prose and more bullet points and tick boxes. References have been excluded from the main text and gathered at the end of each section under 'Further reading'. The tick boxes allow copies of the relevant pages to be inserted into the woman's hospital records, with the relevant boxes ticked, as a supplementary record of the woman's care during labour.

There are other principles which underpin this handbook. The first is a focus on the management of risk. Some of the chapters and the appendices specifically address risk issues, and other chapters have warning boxes or contain elements designed to help minimize human error. Secondly, although (for the sake of simplicity) the chapters are mostly named after clinical conditions and processes, the woman is always at the centre of care – it is the individual woman rather than the condition that should be the focus. Thirdly, the book is addressed to both doctors and midwives, emphasizing the team approach. Also, normal and abnormal labour are regarded as a continuum.

Clinical practice constantly changes as new evidence emerges, and every effort has been made to keep this third edition of *The Labour Ward Handbook* as up to date as possible. I hope that it will facilitate an evidence-based but also holistic approach to care in labour.

Acknowledgements

This book is a compendium of best practice distilled from a variety of sources, including research publications, textbooks, the Cochrane Library, guidelines produced by the UK National Institute for Clinical and Health Excellence (NICE), by postgraduate medical colleges in the UK, Australia, Canada, USA and France, and by specialist societies, and the labour ward protocols of various hospitals, along with my own personal experience.

The book has its origins in guidelines that I compiled for the Royal Oldham Hospital decades ago, with the support of the obstetric, midwifery, anaesthetic, paediatric and administrative staff of that hospital.

For the second edition, I had the benefit of working with teams of obstetricians, anaesthetists, midwives, operating department practitioners and clinical support workers at St Mary's Hospital, Manchester.

The contributions of all are acknowledged gratefully.

About the Author

Leroy C Edozien is a medical doctor and Doctor of Law. His qualifications include degrees in Basic Medical Sciences (BSc, MSc), Medicine (MB BS) and Law (LLB, MPhil, PhD) from the Universities of Ibadan, London and Glasgow, and membership of UK, Irish and West African postgraduate medical colleges (FRCOG, MRCPI FWACS). He holds certificates in Medical Education and Public Policy Analysis from the Royal College of Physicians and the London School of Economics and Political Science respectively.

A former Consultant Obstetrician and Gynaecologist at The Royal Oldham Hospital and at St Mary's Hospital, Manchester, he served for many years as Director of Clinical Audit and Risk Management for Central Manchester teaching hospitals and as Lead for Reproductive Health and Childbirth at the Greater Manchester Comprehensive Research Network. He undertook assignments pertaining to clinical standards and patient safety for the Royal College of Obstetricians and Gynaecologists, National Patient Safety Agency, National Institute of Health and Care Excellence and the National Institute of Health Research. He has served as a medico-legal expert in courts in the UK, Ireland and Australia.

He received a UK national clinical excellence award in 2008 (renewed 2013) for his work as a consultant in Obstetrics and Gynaecology and an authority in Clinical Governance. Final year students at the University of Manchester honoured him as an 'Exceptional Role Model' in 2009.

He was President, North of England Obstetrical and Gynaecological Society 2010; Chairman, British Society of Biopsychosocial Obstetrics and Gynaecology 2014–17; President, International Society of Psychosomatic Obstetrics and Gynaecology 2019–22. He is currently Professor and Director, Institute of Advanced Clinical Sciences Education, University of Medical Sciences, Ondo City

The second edition of *The Labour Ward Handbook* was Highly Commended and shortlisted for the British Medical Association (BMA) Book of the Year 2010.

Abbreviations

The following list includes those abbreviations used frequently in this book as well as those whose use is acceptable in written records:

ALT	alanine aminotransferase
APH	antepartum haemorrhage
APTT	activated partial thromboplastin time
ARDS	adult respiratory distress syndrome
ARM	artificial rupture of fetal membranes
bd	twice daily
BLS	basic life support
BP	blood pressure
CNST	Clinical Negligence Scheme for Trusts
COVID-19	Coronavirus disease 2019
CPR	cardiopulmonary resuscitation
CRP	C-reactive protein
CS	caesarean section
CSF	cerebrospinal fluid
CTG	cardiotocograph
CVP	central venous pressure
DDAVP	desmopressin acetate
DIC	disseminated intravascular coagulopathy
DVT	deep venous thrombosis
ECG	electrocardiography
ECV	external cephalic version
EUA	examination under anaesthetic
EWS	early warning score
FBC	full blood count
FBS	fetal blood sampling
FDP	fibrin degradation product
FFP	fresh frozen plasma
FH	fetal heart
FISH	fluorescence in situ hybridization
FSE	fetal scalp electrode
GBS	group B haemolytic streptococci
[Hb]	haemoglobin concentration
HDU	high-dependency unit
HELLP	haemolysis, elevated liver enzymes, low platelets
HIV	human immunodeficiency virus
HVS	high vaginal swab
IM	(or im) intramuscular
IOL	induction of labour
ITP	immune thrombocytopenic purpura
ITU	intensive therapy unit
IUGR	intrauterine growth restriction

IV	(or iv) intravenous
IVH	intraventricular haemorrhage
LFT	liver function tests
LMWH	low-molecular-weight heparin
MAP	mean arterial pressure
MRSA	Methicillin-resistant *Staphylococcus aureus*
NSAID	non-steroidal anti-inflammatory drug
NTD	neural tube defect
ODA	operating department assistant
OP	occipito-posterior
PDS	polydioxanone sulphate sutures
PPH	postpartum haemorrhage
PROM	prelabour rupture of fetal membranes
PT	prothrombin time
pv	per vaginum
qds	four times daily
RCA	Royal College of Anaesthetists
RCM	Royal College of Midwives
RCOG	Royal College of Obstetricians and Gynaecologists
RDS	respiratory distress syndrome
Rh	rhesus
SBAR	situation, background, assessment, recommendation (a framework for effective communication)
SC	(or sc) subcutaneous
SCBU	special-care baby unit
SLF	systemic lupus erythematosus
SpR	specialist registrar
SROM	spontaneous rupture of fetal membranes
ST	specialty trainee
tds	three times daily
TED	thromboembolism-deterrent stockings
U/E	urea and electrolytes
VE	vaginal examination
V/Q	ventilation–perfusion scan
VTE	venous thromboembolism
vWF	von Willebrand Factor

Glossary

Abnormal lie: Any lie other than longitudinal.

Advance decision: A declaration by a competent person stating what treatment should not be given if the patient loses the capacity to make decisions for themselves.

Anti-Xa assay: Test used to monitor heparin therapy. It measures the Xa inhibitory activity of heparin.

Arterial line: A cannula inserted into a peripheral artery (commonly the radial or brachial artery).

Bishop score: A composite of five indices (station; position; consistency; effacement; and dilation of the cervix) used to predict whether labour can be readily induced.

Central venous pressure (CVP): Pressure in the superior vena cava or right atrium. This is used as a guide to fluid balance in critically ill women and for monitoring circulatory collapse.

Chorionicity: The number of placentas in a multiple pregnancy – with a single shared placenta or one each.

Cleidotomy: Intentional fracture of the baby's collar bone to facilitate delivery.

Clotting (or coagulation) profile: This usually comprises prothrombin time (PT), activated partial thromboplastin time (APTT), fibrinogen and fibrinogen degradation products (FDP).

D-dimer: A protein that is released into the circulation during the process of fibrin blood clot breakdown. D-dimer present in the circulation is used as an indicator of a blood clot being formed and broken down somewhere in the body. D-dimer levels in pregnancy are higher than in the non-pregnant state.

Dystocia: Dysfunctional labour.

Falx cerebri: A structure formed by two leaves of dura, along the sagittal suture.

Fifths palpable: The number of fifths of the baby's head palpable above the pelvic brim. This corresponds to the number of finger breadths palpable above the symphysis pubis. When the head is 'engaged', the bony presenting part (i.e. with the caput excluded) is at the level of the ischial spines and the baby's head is 1/5 to 2/5 palpable abdominally.

Instrumental delivery: Vacuum-assisted (ventouse) or forceps delivery.

Ischial spines: A bony landmark in the pelvis; used to express the level of descent of the baby's head.

Malpresentation: Abnormal presentation – any presentation other than cephalic.

Partogram: Graphic documentation of events in labour.

Patient group direction: A document that allows a registered healthcare professional (normally a nurse or midwife) to supply or administer a prescription-only medicine to a patient without the drug having been prescribed by a doctor.

Plasma substitute: Infusion used to expand and maintain blood volume. Gelofusine and Haemaccel are gelatine of bovine origin. They are recommended in this book since they have no effect on haemostasis. Maize starch products (e.g. Hespan) and hydrolysed starch (Dextran) inhibit clotting.

Rhesus isoimmunization: A condition arising from incompatibility of Rh blood groups in mother and baby.

Tocolysis: Therapeutic arrest of uterine contractions.

Tocolytic: A drug used to stop uterine contractions.

Ventouse delivery: Vacuum-assisted delivery.

Bleep/crash calls

BLEEPS

Obstetric ST (first on call) ....
Obstetric ST (second on call) ....
Paediatric ST (first on call) ....
Paediatric ST (second on call) ....
Anaesthetic ST ....
Anaesthetic assistant: ....

EMERGENCIES

Crash calls for obstetric, paediatric and anaesthetic specialist registrar (SpR)

Obstetrics: ....

Ask for the appropriate doctor to be bleeped urgently. State the place (e.g. delivery suite and room number).

Paediatrics: ....

Request the second-on paediatrician urgently. State the place (e.g. delivery suite and room number).

Anaesthetics ....

State the place (e.g. delivery suite).
Note: If more than one of the specialties is required, it is not necessary to make more than one call. Bleep .... and ask for an urgent call to go out to the appropriate specialties. State the place (e.g. delivery suite and room number).

Cardiac arrest

State the place (e.g. delivery suite and room number).

Fire

Activate the fire alarm. Dial ....
    Wait for the call to be acknowledged. Proceed appropriately with the fire drill, as instructed at the annual fire lecture.

PART I

Approach to care

'... a shift in attention from what is done to patients to what is accomplished for them'
Committee on Quality of Healthcare in America. Institute of Medicine.
Crossing the Quality Chasm: A New Health System for the 21st Century.
Washington, DC: National Academy Press, 2001:44

DOI: 10.1201/9781315099897-1

The biopsychosocial approach to care of the woman in labour

1

Intrapartum care should take account of not only biological but also psychological and social factors. Together, these factors have a significant impact on clinical outcomes and on a woman's wellbeing and her perceptions of childbirth. These perceptions influence the physical and psychological health of the woman, her bonding with the baby and family relationships. A positive experience of childbirth reinforces the woman's confidence in herself and lays a good foundation for family health and future childbearing. A negative birth experience is associated with inhibition of breastfeeding, post-traumatic stress disorder, fear of birth, delay in having another baby, stress in the next pregnancy and maternal request for a planned caesarean delivery in the absence of medical indications.

By adopting a biopsychosocial model of intrapartum care, doctors and midwives can enhance the birth experience of women under their care and achieve optimal clinical outcomes while also securing psychological wellbeing.

The model of care espoused in this book comprises provision of the following:

- Clinical care
- Information (biomedical, behavioural, sociocultural)
- Support (social, cultural, emotional and psychological)

These domains are also captured in the intrapartum care quality statements issued by the UK National Institute for Health and Care Excellence (NICE) – see Box 1.

BOX 1   LIST OF NICE INTRAPARTUM CARE QUALITY STATEMENTS

Statement 1. Women at low risk of complications during labour are given the choice of all birth settings and information about local birth outcomes.

Statement 2. Women in established labour have one-to-one care and support from an assigned midwife.

Statement 3. Women at low risk of complications do not have cardiotocography as part of the initial assessment of labour.

Statement 4. Women at low risk of complications who have cardiotocography because of concern arising from intermittent auscultation have the cardiotocograph removed if the trace is normal for 20 minutes.

Statement 5. Women at low risk of complications are not offered amniotomy or oxytocin if labour is progressing normally.

Statement 6. Women do not have the cord clamped earlier than 1 minute after the birth unless there is concern about cord integrity or the baby's heartbeat.

Statement 7. Women have skin-to-skin contact with their babies after the birth.

DOI: 10.1201/9781315099897-2

The needs of each woman in labour should be accorded PRECEDENCE (see Box 2).

**BOX 2   COMPONENTS OF A BIOPSYCHOSOCIAL
MODEL OF INTRAPARTUM CARE**

P - Person-centred care; culturally sensitive care
R - Relief of pain: optimal, holistic
E - Environment: home or 'home-away-from-home'
C - Continuous midwifery support
E - Education: prelabour and intrapartum
D - Dysfunctional labour optimally managed
E - Empathy; compassionate care
N - Information giving, during and after labour
C - Consent; informed choice; involvement in decision-making
E - Engagement of partner

P – Person-centred care takes into consideration the woman's personal preferences, cultural traditions, values and beliefs. The woman should be constructively engaged in decision-making about her care.

R – Relief of pain. The degree of pain felt or perceived by a woman in labour is influenced by cultural expectations, emotions and state of mind in labour. Encourage ambulation, relaxation techniques like breathing exercises, immersion in water, distraction or visual imagery, and massage.

E – Environment. As much as practicable, the delivery suite should have the feel of 'home-away-from-home'.

C – Continuous presence of a supportive companion; the most important intervention proven to be beneficial in labour.

E – Education. Perinatal education strengthens the woman's 'sense of coherence', a measure of her confidence in deploying personal attributes to achieve optimal birth outcome.

D – Dysfunctional labour should be optimally managed. It is not just a mechanical issue: may be caused or prevented by biopsychosocial factors and may cause psychological problems. (See Chapter 12, Management of the first stage of labour.)

E – Empathy. Nurture a culture of respect for a woman undergoing an intense life experience. The woman should be listened to and cared for with compassion.

N – Information. The labouring woman should be given adequate information regarding the progress of labour and about every intervention and every procedure offered or carried out. She should be given as much information as she desires and in a language she understands. The information should also be provided to the partner who is providing emotional support to the woman. Concise and clear explanations of *what* is being proposed (or what is happening), *why* this is necessary, *how* it will be done and *when* it will be done are generally adequate – but often not provided.

C – Consent. The pregnant woman, like any other recipient of medical treatment, has the right to determine what treatment to accept or to decline. In exercising the right to self-determination in pregnancy care, the woman relies on the information provided by the doctor or midwife, and the right cannot be said to have been upheld if the woman is not in a position to make an informed choice. See Appendix: Guidance for obtaining consent to treatment.

E – Engage fathers. Fathers see themselves as much more than just passive supporters for their partners; they want to be authentically engaged but are often regarded as 'not-patient and not-visitor'. Their expectation of active engagement leads to profound trauma where events do not go well (clinical events or dehumanizing behaviour from staff). Doctors and midwives who adopt a family-centred approach are more likely to engage fathers than those who see only the pregnant woman as their concern. Separate from their role in supporting the woman in labour, men have their own anxieties and needs as they play out this role. Witnessing a birth that is traumatic, or perceived as traumatic, can leave the father with long-term psychological problems.

Sometimes the midwife or doctor may find it difficult to distinguish the intentions of a man who is simply being keen or concerned about his partner's wellbeing and their baby's safety from those of a man who is manifesting a controlling streak. Good communication skills will help to resolve the dilemma.

1.1 ASSESSING WOMEN'S SATISFACTION WITH INTRAPARTUM CARE

Tools have been developed for assessing women's satisfaction with their care in labour. Some of these are listed as follows.

- Labour and Delivery Satisfaction Index (LADSI)
- Perceptions of Care Adjective Checklist (PCACL-R)
- Intrapartal care in relation to WHO recommendations (IC-WHO)
- Patient Perception Score (PPS, designed for operative births)
- Questionnaire to assess clients' satisfaction (CliSQ)
- Intrapartal-Specific QPP-questionnaire (QPP-I)
- Six Simple Questions (SSQ)
- Maternal Satisfaction for Caesarean Section (MSCS)
- Consumer Satisfaction Questionnaire (CSQ)

'Women want good clinical outcomes for themselves and their babies, but they also want to be treated humanely, with dignity and with respect for their right to self-determination. A biopsychosocial approach to intrapartum care combines the best available evidence with person-centred care to achieve the best clinical and psychological outcomes for the woman, her partner, and their baby.'

Leroy C Edozien
(Biopsychosocial factors in intrapartum care. In: Edozien & O'Brien,
Biopsychosocial Factors in Obstetrics and Gynaecology. Cambridge:
Cambridge University Press, 2017)

Communication between care providers

2

For efficient delivery of care, it is important that lines of communication be well defined. The consultant under whose care the mother is booked is ultimately responsible for her care. For each shift on the delivery suite, one midwife of appropriate seniority and experience will be designated coordinator and will be responsible for coordinating the work of the delivery suite and providing necessary support, guidance and supervision of midwives and medical staff. The coordinator should be informed regularly of each mother's progress. The names of the coordinator and the obstetric, anaesthetic and paediatric medical staff on duty should be on the designated notice board.

The lines of communication for the midwife are through the coordinator and the resident medical staff. However, any midwife or other member of staff who has concerns about a woman's care may contact the ST or consultant (obstetric or anaesthetic) directly.

All members of the duty obstetric team should ensure that they are readily accessible and available at all times.

2.1 EARLY IDENTIFICATION AND COMMUNICATION OF RISK

Failure to escalate or act upon risk was a contributory factor in one-half of the perinatal deaths investigated in the 2018 *Each Baby Counts* project.

For women at high risk, a signed plan of management should be made antenatally and written in the handheld and hospital records. Early identification of risk factors, anticipation of problems and effective communication are key factors for good management.

If a non-duty consultant has an interest in the management of a particular woman then this should be marked clearly in the case notes; the senior midwife or ST will need to contact this consultant when the woman is admitted and if problems arise afterwards.

All high-risk women admitted to the labour ward must be seen by the doctor on duty as soon as possible.

The specialty trainee/registrar should be informed immediately of any untoward problems and of any of the following conditions (note that this is not an exhaustive list):

- APH
- PPH
- Malpresentation
- Cord prolapse/cord presentation
- Severe pre-eclampsia/eclampsia

DOI: 10.1201/9781315099897-3

- Multiple pregnancy
- Preterm labour
- PROM
- Abnormal fetal heart rate
- Diabetes mellitus
- Cardiac disease
- Intrauterine death
- Large baby
- Previous CS
- Any pregnancy identified as high-risk in the case notes

If there is any delay in response in cases such as prolapsed cord or if the registrar is unavailable because of another emergency, then the consultant on call should be called immediately.

It is recommended that the consultant should be physically present for the following:

- Eclampsia
- Maternal collapse (resulting from placental abruption, septic shock or other abnormality)
- CS for major placenta praevia
- PPH of more than 1.5 L where the haemorrhage is continuing and a massive obstetric haemorrhage protocol has been instigated
- Return to theatre – laparotomy

2.2 HANDOVER

There should be a personal handover of patient care at the shift/on-call changeover of both midwifery and medical staff. There should be ward rounds at 0830, 1300 and 1700. Where there is no resident consultant, there should be, as a minimum, a telephone review with the non-resident consultant at 2200.

There should be a professional approach to the ward rounds – which means no distractions such as telephone or side conversations. At each ward round, but particularly at the morning and evening rounds, there should be an assessment of the number and experience of the available workforce, identification of any threats to the service (e.g. non-availability of cots in the neonatal unit) and a review of patient safety incidents from the outgoing shift. The handover offers an opportunity to identify risks, make contingency plans and develop shared mental models for the challenges ahead. This helps to maintain situational awareness. Lack of situational awareness was a contributory factor in 47% of the perinatal deaths investigated in the 2018 *Each Baby Counts* project.

The maternity unit should devise a Structured Multidisciplinary Intershift Handover (SMITH) tool to facilitate team communications and handover between shifts (See Further reading on p. 18).

2.3 COMMUNICATION WITH ANAESTHETISTS

In anticipation of events, the anaesthetist should be informed at an early stage of any of the following:

- APH
- Twin pregnancy in labour
- Breech vaginal delivery

- Previous CS
- Woman at risk of PPH
- Pre-eclampsia
- Obese patient who may require operative intervention
- Medical conditions such as diabetes, sickle cell and heart disease
- History of anaphylaxis

'Provision of obstetric care is by its nature multidisciplinary. The team, which includes obstetricians, anaesthetists, neonatologists, midwives, theatre staff, anaesthetic assistants and others, has to be able to work closely under stress in dynamic situations. To ensure that teams can function effectively in this environment, they need to train together and have the appropriate infrastructure and necessary resources in place to deliver a high-quality service.'

Royal College of Anaesthetists. *Guidelines for the Provision of Anaesthetic Services.* **Chapter 9: Guidelines for the Provision of Anaesthesia Services for an Obstetric Population 2022. RCA, January 2022**

'Failings in communication and lack of teamwork between obstetric, midwifery and anaesthetic staff were a recurring theme and clearly contributed to critical delays in the care of the mothers, with devastating outcomes for their otherwise healthy, full term babies.'

RCOG. *Each Baby Counts project.* **Themed report on anaesthetic care, including lessons identified from Each Baby Counts babies born 2015 to 2017. RCOG, July 2018**

'A good working relationship between the multidisciplinary team (midwives, medical, ancillary, managerial staff) and the women in their care is crucial to ensure optimal birth outcomes. This is best achieved with a team approach, based on mutual respect, a shared philosophy of care and a clear organizational structure for both midwives and medical staff with explicit and transparent lines of communication. Clear, accurate and respectful communication between all team members and each discipline is essential, as well as with women and their families.'

Royal College of Obstetricians and Gynaecologists, Royal College of Midwives, Royal College of Anaesthetists, Royal College of Paediatrics and Child Health. *Safer Childbirth: Minimum Standards for the Organisation and Delivery of Care in Labour, Report of a Working Party.* **London: RCOG Press, 2007:10**

Documentation

3

Poor record keeping was a contributory factor in 23% of the perinatal deaths reviewed in the 2018 *Each Baby Counts* report.

Regardless of whether electronic records (contemporaneous or retrospective) or paper records are used, the care given should be documented carefully and thoughtfully.

For electronic systems, log in with your own identification details, and log out after documentation.

All examinations, results, clinical communications and maternal requests should be documented accurately in the labour notes, partogram and CTG trace as appropriate.

Use abbreviations sparingly, and only those in standard use (e.g. CS, FH).

Consent for examination, CS and other interventions must follow standard policy and practice (see Appendix).

Every operative delivery should be written up in detail, with the date, time, indication(s), findings and any complications stated clearly. Instructions for postoperative care should be itemized. Proformas for CS, instrumental vaginal delivery and repair of perineal tears help to raise the quality of documentation.

The time of decision to perform a CS, and the degree of urgency, should be documented. The time of commencement of CS, i.e. 'knife to skin', should be recorded in the theatre logbook.

For paper records:

All entries must be clearly signed, dated and timed (use the 24-hour clock). Illegible signatures are not acceptable. Always print your name and grade below your signature.

Every loose-leaf sheet in the notes must have patient identification. The responsibility for this rests with the first person who writes on that page.

Before filing any results, check that they belong to the correct patient, annotate any action required or taken, and append your signature.

Every CTG trace should bear the patient's identification label and the date and time of commencement and completion. The maternal pulse should be recorded regularly on the trace (not just at the beginning), along with any key events in care. Any loss of contact or discontinuation should be annotated on the trace.

Sign and date all CTGs, and file them securely with the clinical records.

The standard setting of 1 cm/min should not be altered on the CTG monitor.

Never try to alter existing notes. If corrections are necessary, draw a line through the incorrect entry and sign and date the additional note.

All midwifery records must comply with standards set by the Nursing and Midwifery Council.

The statutory limitation on obstetric litigation is not until the child is 21 years of age, so notes relating to pregnancy care must be maintained intact for this duration.

DOI: 10.1201/9781315099897-4

Admission to, and discharge home from, the delivery suite

4

4.1 ADMISSION

The admission process affords an opportunity to reassess the woman's risk status and to plan her care accordingly. Deficiencies pertaining to risk recognition were a contributory factor in 3 out of every 4 perinatal deaths investigated in the 2018 *Each Baby Counts* project.

The initial assessment will be by a named midwife to whom the woman has been introduced. Where indicated (see Chapter 2), the admitting midwife should refer to the doctor on duty, without delay. The antenatal clinic records and records of any admissions in the pregnancy should be reviewed and any special instructions noted. A plan of care should be devised with the woman, building on wishes and plans agreed during antenatal care. This plan should be flexible, and subject to review during labour. Document the reason for admission, the findings on assessment and the plan of care.

4.2 DISCHARGE

An experienced midwife may discharge a woman home when labour has been excluded, provided that the following criteria are met:

- Normal, uneventful pregnancy at 37–40 weeks
- Normal medical history
- Normal maternal observations
- Normal admission CTG, where this test is indicated
- No abnormal vaginal loss
- Normal vaginal examination with no indication that labour has established
- Intact membranes
- First referral to delivery suite in this pregnancy
- Woman is happy to go home
- Follow-up appointment is given

A woman who presents with deviations from the aforementioned criteria should be referred to the doctor on call for further assessment. A woman not wishing to go home may be transferred to the antenatal ward.

DOI: 10.1201/9781315099897-5

Learning from clinical incidents

5

The labour ward should have formal systems for learning from clinical incidents and for sharing lessons learned. Apart from structures and processes, such as the multidisciplinary labour ward forum and mechanisms for reporting incidents, a culture of safety should be nurtured.

5.1 WHAT IS A CLINICAL INCIDENT?

A clinical incident (also known as a patient safety incident, adverse event or critical incident) is an untoward event that happened to a woman during or as a result of care or treatment and that has caused, or could cause, an adverse outcome.

All incidents on the trigger list, and any others that, in the opinion of the ward manager, fall within the scope of this definition, must be reported as detailed later.

It is not practicable to provide an exhaustive list of clinical incidents, but the more common examples are:

- Maternal death
- Stillbirth
- Neonatal death
- Low Apgar score: <6 at 5 minutes
- Undiagnosed breech
- Shoulder dystocia
- Major PPH ($\geq$1000 mL)
- Postpartum [Hb] <8 g/dL
- Eclampsia or other fits
- Unexpected transfer to neonatal unit, including neonatal seizures
- Medication errors
- Significant infections
- Loss of clinical materials (e.g. swabs)
- Unavailability of health record
- Return to theatre
- Third- and fourth-degree tears
- Readmission of either mother or baby
- Unavailability of any facility or equipment, including neonatal unit cots
- Misdiagnosis of antenatal screening tests
- Unplanned home birth
- Cord pH <7.05
- Maternal transfer to ITU
- Maternal resuscitation
- Injury to bladder or other organs

DOI: 10.1201/9781315099897-6

- First stage of labour >17 hours
- Second stage of labour >3 hours
- Birth injury
  - Subdural haematoma or tear of falx cerebri
  - Any fracture (e.g. skull, clavicle, long bone)
  - Any paralysis (e.g. brachial plexus injury)
- Major congenital abnormalities first detected at delivery
- Any event considered to be serious, regardless of outcome

5.2 WHY DO WE NEED CLINICAL INCIDENT ANALYSIS?

By continual review of clinical incidents, we could learn lessons, improve care and reduce risks to women and babies:

- Near misses are an important source of information to prevent such events happening again.
- Identification of common themes can help to predict and prevent future incidents.
- Early warning signs can be picked up.

We can promote a culture of learning and enquiry and help all members of the multidisciplinary team to reflect on their practice and make changes as necessary. The principle is not to blame or shame but to promote active learning and improve the quality of care.

Clinical incidents are commonly due to inadequacies in the system rather than the fault of an individual. Analysis of incidents will be used to determine how the system can be improved, not to punish the individual. The analysis will be used to identify unexpected events and those with poor outcomes that may need further investigation. Once risk factors or patterns emerge, we can focus on prevention and education. Information could alert line managers to possible weaknesses in systems of work.

Clinical incident analysis will provide an archive of facts for possible use in medico-legal cases.

5.3 REPORTING CLINICAL INCIDENTS

Incidents should be reported using the hospital's incident reporting form (electronic or paper) and in line with the hospital's risk management strategy.

5.4 LEARNING FROM CLINICAL INCIDENTS

In addition to use of the incident reporting system, the unit will identify clinical incidents and risks through prospective risk assessments, clinical audit, complaints and claims. Reported incidents will be analysed and investigated as stipulated in the hospital's risk management strategy. Periodic summaries of reported incidents will be provided. It is more important to report what changes have been implemented and what demonstrable benefits have resulted from reported incidents.

Lessons learned from the identification and treatment of risk should be shared with other parts of the hospital/trust and with the wider community as may be appropriate, through channels such as multidisciplinary team meetings, ward meetings, safety alerts, newsletters, intranet and educational meetings.

The labour ward/maternity unit should have a risk register that lists major risks and what control measures are in place or planned. A maternity 'dashboard' is also a useful device for monitoring progress with risk control.

5.5 CONFIDENTIALITY

Practitioners are expected to respect the confidentiality of their patients and colleagues when undertaking a review. Information will be always handled in a way that protects patients' confidentiality and in keeping with the Data Protection Act. Anonymous reporting is preferable to concealment. Incidents or near misses may be reported anonymously or (preferably) confidentially to the ward manager, the consultant or the risk management midwife.

Transfer of care between professionals

6

6.1 BACKGROUND

This guidance stems from recommendations by various bodies concerned with quality of care:

- The NHS Litigation Authority (NHSLA) – now operating under the name NHS Resolution – standards called for clear arrangements concerning which professional is responsible for the patient's care at all times.
- The *Confidential Enquiries into Stillbirths and Deaths in Infancy (CESDI)* and its successor bodies emphasized the importance of adequate arrangements for transfer of patients between units.
- The Royal Colleges and the UK National Institute of Health and Care Excellence (NICE) state that explicit lines of communication between professionals are crucial to optimization of birth outcomes.
- Poor intra- or inter-professional communication was a contributory factor in 43% of the perinatal deaths analysed in the 2018 *Each Baby Counts* project.

6.2 HANDOVER BY CLINICAL STAFF

There should be a formal handover on the ward at 0830, 1300 and 1700 on weekdays and at 0900 at weekends. Each unit will have its own arrangements for night-time handovers. The handover takes priority over other, non-emergency clinical duties. Units are encouraged to have their own Structured Multidisciplinary Intershift Handover (SMITH) tool.

The baton bleep should be handed over personally to the incoming person – it is unacceptable to leave the bleep at the ward station or reception.

Transitions of care between individual practitioners and between clinical areas should follow a formal local protocol. The outgoing practitioner should summarize in writing the clinical status of the woman (including the early warning score (EWS), where applicable) and itemize what needs to be done. The SBAR (situation, background, assessment, recommendation) framework is recommended for communicating transfers of care.

6.3 TRANSFER OF EMERGENCIES FROM PRIMARY CARE

Emergency transfers to the labour ward can be made at any time by the GP or community midwife after discussion with the medical or midwifery staff. The coordinator must be informed. Some referrals will be

DOI: 10.1201/9781315099897-7

more appropriate to the maternity day assessment unit or the early pregnancy assessment unit and should be directed accordingly.

6.4 TRANSFER BETWEEN HOSPITALS WITH THE FETUS IN UTERO

- All transfers in or out must be with the prior approval of the consultant obstetrician.
- If there is a good chance that the baby will need to be delivered in the next 48 hours, then availability of a cot in the neonatal unit of the receiving hospital must be confirmed before transfer.
- Where indicated, prophylactic steroids should be given before transfer in or out.
- Where indicated, a tocolytic should be given before transfer in or out.
- Appropriate personnel should accompany the woman. The coordinating midwife and the consultant obstetrician will determine the appropriate personnel for each case.
- Do not transfer (or accept a transfer) if any of the following apply:
  - Uncontrolled vaginal bleeding
  - Cervix >4 cm dilated
  - Three or more uterine contractions in 10 minutes.
- A letter and a copy (not the original) of the notes should accompany the woman.
- Results of relevant investigations should be recorded in the notes or telephoned through to the receiving hospital as soon as they are available.
- Ensure that the woman is appropriately dressed and kept warm.
- For women transferred from another hospital, an MRSA screen should be performed on admission.

6.5 TRANSFER OF CARE BETWEEN CONSULTANTS

When a patient is referred to a special or subspecialty clinic, there should be a referral letter indicating whether this is an outright transfer or a request for opinion only.

For emergency admission of unbooked patients, the woman is under the consultant on call at the time of admission, unless she has an unfinished clinical episode under another consultant, in which case she remains under that consultant's care. A clinical episode, in this context, finishes when a discharge letter has been written.

6.6 TRANSFER BACK TO THE COMMUNITY OR GP CARE

Follow-up plans/arrangements should always be specified in the case notes (hospital and handheld) and in discharge letters. If no follow-up appointment has been arranged, then this should be stated in a discharge letter.

Following a stillbirth, miscarriage or termination for fetal anomaly, the GP, community midwife and health visitor must be informed immediately (see also Chapter 91).

Where it has been arranged for a patient to be followed up by the community midwife, this should be documented in the case notes and in the diary kept on the unit.

6.7 TRANSFER TO ICU AND HDU

6.7.1 Who transfers?

A patient may be transferred to ICU or HDU at the request of the consultant obstetrician/gynaecologist, consultant anaesthetist or anaesthetic registrar. All transfers to ITU must be discussed first with the consultant anaesthetist in charge.

6.8 WHO IS IN CHARGE WHILE THE WOMAN IS IN ICU OR HDU?

A patient in ICU is primarily under the care of the consultant anaesthetist, but the consultant obstetrician remains responsible for the obstetric care. Any woman admitted into ICU must be seen daily by the obstetric team.

The duty consultant obstetrician is primarily responsible for women in Maternity HDU.

The consultant obstetrician/gynaecologist is primarily responsible for the care of his or her patient transferred to the Surgical HDU.

6.9 RETURN TO DELIVERY SUITE FROM ICU

The consultant obstetrician and consultant obstetric anaesthetist should be involved in the decision to transfer/accept the transfer from ICU to delivery suite, and one of them should see the woman before she is transferred. The SBAR framework is recommended for a structured transfer.

Both the physical and the psychological needs of the woman should be addressed.

If possible, transfers from the ICU to the delivery suite at night should be avoided.

Reviewing what happened

7

It is often helpful if the newly delivered mother has an opportunity to discuss her experience with a professional who was involved in her care. Events are reviewed and, where necessary, issues are clarified.

The review provides the opportunity for the mother to:

- Ask questions
- Express her feelings, e.g. pleasure, gratitude, fear, anger, confusion or other emotions
- Understand the reasons for unmet expectations
- Be reassured of her success and her achievement
- Be given explanations and apologies, as may be necessary
- Plan for future pregnancies

The review should be held at a mutually convenient time before discharge. The format of the review is not prescriptive. It should be a listening and sharing activity, not a counselling activity.

A summary of the following should be recorded in the postnatal records:

- Date and time of meeting, and who attended
- Matter discussed
- Questions asked
- Unresolved issues, if any
- Further action required

Where difficulties are experienced, support and advice should be sought from a ward manager, supervisor or consultant or from the hospital's patient advice and liaison service.

Some women may prefer to speak with a midwife or obstetrician who was not involved in the delivery.

If a complaint is imminent, then the hospital's complaints policy should be followed.

DOI: 10.1201/9781315099897-8

Further reading for Part I

Communication

Dadiz R, Weinschreider J, Schriefer J, Arnold C, Greves CD, Crosby EC, Wang H, Pressman EK, Guillet R. Interdisciplinary simulation-based training to improve delivery room communication. *Simul Healthc.* 2013;8(5):279–91. doi: 10.1097/SIH.0b013e31829543a3

Edozien LC. Structured multidisciplinary intershift handover (SMITH): a tool for promoting safer intrapartum care. *J Obstet Gynaecol.* 2011;31(8):683–686. doi:10.3109/01443615.2011.595518

Royal College of Obstetricians and Gynaecologists. *Each Baby Counts: 2020 Final Progress Report.* London: RCOG, 2021

Sundgren NC, Kelly FC, Weber EM, et al. Improving communication between obstetric and neonatology teams for high-risk deliveries: A quality improvement project. *BMJ Open Qual.* 2017;6:e000095. doi: 10.1136/bmjoq-2017-000095

Sundgren NC, Suresh GK. How do obstetric and neonatology teams communicate prior to high-risk deliveries? *Am J Perinatol.* 2018;35(1):10–15. doi: 10.1055/s-0037-1604391

Documentation

General Medical Council. *Good Medical Practice Knowledge Skills and Performance*, paragraph 19–21. GMC, 2013

Nursing and Midwifery Council. *The Code: Professional Standards of Practice and Behaviour for Nurses, Midwives and Nursing Associates.* NMC, 2015; updated 2018

Royal College of Obstetricians and Gynaecologists. *Each Baby Counts: 2020 Final Progress Report.* RCOG, 2021

Clinical incident reporting

Hewitt T, Chreim S, Forster, A. Incident reporting systems: A comparative study of two hospital divisions. *Arch Public Health.* 2016;74:34. doi: 10.1186/s13690-016-0146-8

Jäger C, Mohr G, Gökcimen K, Navarini A, Schwendimann R, Müller S. Critical incident reporting over time: A retrospective, descriptive analysis of 5493 cases. *Swiss Med Wkly.* 2021;151:w30098. doi: 10.4414/smw.2021.w30098

Macdonald M, Gosakan R, Cooper AE, Fothergill DJ. Dealing with a serious incident requiring investigation in obstetrics and gynaecology: A training perspective. *Obstet Gynecol.* 2014;16:109–14

DOI: 10.1201/9781315099897-9

PART II

Normal and Low-Risk Labour

'I have stated on numerous occasions that there is no more need to interfere with the course of normally progressing labor than there is to tamper with good digestion, normal respiration, and adequate circulation'.

Montgomery TL. Physiologic considerations in labor and the puerperium.
Am J Obstet Gynecol. 1958;76:706–15

DOI: 10.1201/9781315099897-10

Vaginal examination

8

8.1 BEFORE VAGINAL EXAMINATION

- Consent must be obtained.
- The history should be reviewed.
- Ultrasound scan results should be noted, where applicable.
- Abdominal examination and auscultation should be performed.

8.2 DURING VAGINAL EXAMINATION

- Ensure privacy and dignity.
- Communicate with the woman.
- Be alert to nonverbal cues. This is particularly important for women with past traumatic experiences.

8.3 DETAILS TO BE RECORDED

- Date and time
- Findings on abdominal examination
- Indication for vaginal examination
- Relevant information on condition of external genitalia and vagina
- Cervical effacement (the length of the cervical canal in centimetres)
- Cervical dilatation
- Presentation
- Level of presenting part in relation to ischial spines
- Application to cervix
- Caput
- Moulding:
    - +   Skull bones apposed
    - ++   Reducible overlap of bones
    - +++ Irreducible overlap of bones
- Membranes:
    - Intact or absent
    - Colour and volume of amniotic fluid
- Fetal heart auscultation following procedure
- Findings explained to mother
- Signature and printed name

DOI: 10.1201/9781315099897-11

Intravenous cannulation

9

In the USA, most women presenting in labour undergo intravenous cannulation. In other countries, cannulation is by indication only.

Intravenous cannulation is recommended for patients with:

- Previous PPH
- Grandmultiparity (fifth and subsequent labours)
- Anaemia ([Hb] <10 g/dL)
- Multiple pregnancy
- Previous CS (undergoing a trial of vaginal delivery)
- Meconium-stained amniotic fluid
- High-risk pregnancy, where the likelihood of operative intervention or peripartum haemorrhage is significant

10 mL of blood for group-and-save serum and FBC should be sent to the laboratory. All group-and-save serum samples should be signed by two professionals.

The cannula should be flushed using either 5 mL 0.9% saline or 5 mL (50 IU) heparin sodium. Use the latter if the cannula is in place for more than 48 hours.

Syntocinon (oxytocin) infusion may be commenced as per patient group direction when:

- Induction of labour has been agreed previously by an obstetrician.
- There is slow progress and the obstetrician on call has confirmed that labour should be augmented.

All indications, discussions and agreement should be documented. In the event of PPH occurring, an infusion of 40 units Syntocinon in 500 mL Hartmann's solution may be commenced while awaiting medical assistance.

No IV fluids other than those indicated on the patient group direction should be given without being prescribed by a doctor.

A giving set that does not contain blood products or lipids can be retained for up to 96 hours without increasing the risk of infection.

- Inspect the cannula insertion site at the beginning of a new shift. Remove the catheter if there are signs of inflammation, blockage or other defect.

DOI: 10.1201/9781315099897-12

Management of normal labour

10

Normal labour will be managed by the midwifery staff. A comprehensive risk assessment should be undertaken when a woman is admitted in labour, and risk is continually assessed during labour.

10.1 CRITERIA FOR NORMAL LABOUR

Normal labour is defined by the presence of all the following criteria:

- Uncomplicated pregnancy (most women will have been booked for midwifery-led care)
- Spontaneous onset of labour at 37–41 weeks' gestation
- Minimum rate of cervical dilation 1 cm/h from diagnosis of established labour
- First admission to labour ward
- Single fetus with engaged head
- Clear amniotic fluid
- Normal maternal observations
- No intrapartum bleeding
- No maternal or fetal distress
- Normal delivery within 1 hour of good expulsive effort
- Intact perineum, first- or second-degree tear or episiotomy
- Third stage lasts for less than 20 minutes following active management
- Immediate postpartum blood loss <500 mL

The doctor should be called to see any woman falling outside these criteria.
    Initial assessment on admission should include the following:

- BP
- Pulse rate
- Respiratory rate
- Temperature
- Urinalysis
- Recording of the fetal heart with a handheld Doppler device
- Abdominal palpation: symphysio–fundal height, presentation, position and fifths palpable (see Glossary)
- Uterine contractions: frequency, duration and strength
- Fetal membranes and, if they are ruptured, colour of amniotic fluid (clear/blood-stained/ meconium-stained)
- MRSA assessment, if indicated and as directed by local policy

DOI: 10.1201/9781315099897-13

Prelabour rupture of membranes at term (37–42 weeks)

11

A woman with suspected spontaneous rupture of membranes and no associated contractions or vaginal bleeding may be assessed (CTG, sterile speculum examination) on the antenatal ward, in the day unit or at triage.

If the woman is bleeding or has uterine contractions, then she should be admitted to the delivery suite. If the CTG is abnormal, the woman must be seen immediately by a doctor.

An experienced midwife may perform a speculum examination provided that the following criteria are met:

- Normal uneventful pregnancy at 37–40 weeks
- Normal fetal heart rate
- No vaginal bleeding
- Consent obtained

If there are no uterine contractions it is not necessary to perform a digital examination.

A vaginal swab should not be taken as a routine, but the clinician can use their judgement to decide when a vaginal swab might give clinically useful information.

If PROM is confirmed, the woman should be advised that:

- The risk of serious neonatal infection is 1 in 100 (compared with 1 in 200 for women with intact membranes).
- 6 of every 10 women with PROM at term will go into labour within 24 hours.
- Induction of labour is appropriate approximately 24 hours after rupture of the membranes.

The mother may be observed on the antenatal ward if PROM is confirmed and the following criteria are met:

- No meconium-stained amniotic fluid
- Cephalic presentation, well-applied to the cervix
- Normal maternal observations
- <24 hours have elapsed since rupture of the membranes

If any of these criteria do not apply, then the obstetrician on call should be informed.

Where PROM is excluded, the discharge protocol should be followed.

DOI: 10.1201/9781315099897-14

11.1 FURTHER MANAGEMENT

Women with confirmed PROM should be offered a choice of expectant management (not exceeding 72 hours) or immediate induction of labour.

The benefits and risks of expectant management versus immediate induction of labour should be discussed, and the agreed plan should be documented. A Cochrane Review detected no differences regarding mode of birth between immediate induction of labour and expectant management – the concern that immediate induction might result in more caesarean and operative births was not supported. Significantly fewer women in the planned management group than those in the expectant management group had chorioamnionitis or endometritis. No difference was seen in terms of neonatal infection, but fewer infants under planned management went to neonatal intensive or special care than did those in expectant management.

If the woman is known to be group B haemolytic streptococcus-positive, labour should be induced immediately, and antibiotics should be prescribed.

11.2 EXPECTANT MANAGEMENT

Await spontaneous onset of labour.

11.2.1 Antibiotics

Antibiotics should not be given in the absence of signs of infection. If there are signs of infection, then prescribe a full course of broad-spectrum IV antibiotics.

11.2.2 When to intervene

If there are any clinical signs suggestive of infection (tachycardia, pyrexia), induce labour.

If observations are normal but labour does not ensue, induce after 12–72 hours (as agreed with the woman).

11.2.3 Induction protocol (see section 41.5 for details)

- Bishop score <5: prostaglandin 1 mg (or 2 mg if nulliparous). Reassess 6 hours later if not in labour.
- Bishop score ≥5: Syntocinon infusion.

11.2.4 Observe the baby

If 18 hours had elapsed since rupture of the membranes, antibiotics should be given.

If labour had not started 24 hours after PROM, the woman should be advised to stay in hospital for at least 12 hours following the birth – so that the baby can be observed for signs of infection. The baby, if asymptomatic, should be observed at 1 hour, 2 hours and then 2-hourly for 10 hours. These observations should include:

- General wellbeing
- Chest movements and nasal flare
- Skin colour, including perfusion, by testing capillary refill
- Feeding
- Muscle tone
- Temperature
- Heart rate and respiration

11.3 ACTIVE MANAGEMENT

Induce with prostaglandin or Syntocinon, as earlier. See Chapter 35 for the protocol for induction of labour.

An alternative, but unlicensed, option is active management with oral or vaginal misoprostol:

- Oral 50 mg, repeated every 4 hours if required, to a maximum of five doses.
- Vaginal 25 µg (50 µg in nulliparous women with Bishop score ≤ 4), followed by 25 µg after 4 and 8 hours.

Uterine rupture following induction of labour with misoprostol has been reported, and the dose stated above should not be exceeded.

Management of the first stage of labour 12

12.1 DIAGNOSIS

It is important to get the diagnosis of labour right since this is the fundamental decision on which all subsequent management is based. Diagnosis is based on painful, regular contractions along with one or more of the following:

- 'Show'
- Spontaneous rupture of membranes
- Cervical effacement and dilatation on vaginal examination >2 cm (primipara) or >3 cm (multipara)

Unwarranted interventions in the latent phase of labour, particularly amniotomy, could convert an otherwise normal labour to an abnormal one.

12.2 MONITORING PROGRESS OF LABOUR

If the woman is in established labour, then her progress and wellbeing should be assessed and managed by her named midwife, who will be aware at all times of the patient's wishes.

Commence partogram and record all maternal and fetal observations.

- Pulse rate should be recorded every hour.
- Record temperature and respiratory rate every 4 hours if apyrexial, but every hour if the woman is pyrexial.
- BP should be recorded at least every half-hour if the woman is hypertensive or having epidural analgesia; in other cases, BP should be recorded every 4 hours.
- Frequency and strength of contractions should be recorded every half-hour.

Descent of the presenting part should be assessed abdominally (fifths palpable) and vaginally (centimetres above or below the ischial spines). Do not rely on vaginal examination only, since caput and moulding may give a false impression of lower descent.

Repeat vaginal examinations at 4-hourly intervals unless there is a reason to examine at shorter intervals.

DOI: 10.1201/9781315099897-15

12.3 BIRTH PLANS

• Check whether she has a birth plan, either written or unwritten.

Birth plans should be respected and supported as much as possible.

If any change in the birth plan becomes necessary, this should be discussed with the mother and a record should be made. Engaging the mother in this way enhances her birth experience.

12.4 SUPPORT PERSON

The continuous presence of a midwife or other support person (partner, friend or family) reduces the likelihood of operative delivery or low Apgar score. It is also associated with a shorter duration of labour and reduced requirement for analgesia.

A link worker should be present if needed or requested.

12.5 POSITIONING

Adoption of the upright position during labour facilitates efficient uterine contractions, shortens the latent phase and reduces the need for analgesia. The woman should be encouraged to move around and adopt whatever position she finds most comfortable during labour.

12.6 NUTRITION

A woman in labour needs energy and should not be starved unless she is likely to require a general anaesthetic. If she is in normal labour, the woman may have a high-carbohydrate/low-fat diet if she wishes.

Fluids may be taken freely in normal labour. When surgery is anticipated, non-particulate, non-fizzy drinks may be taken up to 2 hours before an operation.

Narcotic analgesics delay stomach emptying. If these are used, the woman should avoid food and particulate drinks.

12.7 ANTACIDS (INCLUDING H2-RECEPTOR ANTAGONISTS)

These should not be given routinely to low-risk women. Antacid prophylaxis should be given selectively in labour to women considered to be at high risk for operative intervention.

12.7.1 Dose

Ranitidine 150 mg orally every 6 hours until completion of the third stage. Women who are vomiting, who have had opioid analgesia or who are otherwise unable to take oral medication should be given ranitidine 50 mg IM 6-hourly.

Women not in labour but undergoing a 'crash' CS should have IV ranitidine 50 mg in 20 mL 0.9% saline over 2 minutes and IV metoclopramide 10 mg.

12.8 PAIN RELIEF

The woman should be informed of the various methods of pain relief that are available. The analgesia requested should be administered and documented as per patient group direction.

Breathing, relaxation and massage techniques may be used.

Transcutaneous electrical nerve stimulation (TENS) should not be offered to women in established labour.

12.9 ENTONOX (50% O_2 AND 50% N_2O)

Fully disposable breathing systems should be used. Where this is not available, the Entonox apparatus should include anti-infective filters.

The woman should be informed that it may make her feel nauseous and light-headed.

12.10 OPIOIDS (PETHIDINE, DIAMORPHINE OR OTHER)

The woman should be informed of the side effects: drowsiness, nausea and vomiting in the mother; short-term respiratory depression and drowsiness in the baby.

12.10.1 Pethidine

In established labour, pethidine may be given, in a dose dependent on the woman's weight:

- <60 kg 100 mg IM 3–4-hourly
- >60 kg 150 mg IM 3–4-hourly

An antiemetic (e.g. metoclopramide 10 mg IM) should be given with the first dose of pethidine.

12.10.2 Diamorphine

Compared with pethidine, this is associated with a higher level of pain relief, less maternal vomiting and a lower incidence of low 1-minute Apgar scores.

12.10.3 Remifentanil PCA

An ultrashort-acting synthetic opioid

- Off-label use.
- Not as effective as epidural but a useful alternative where epidural is contraindicated or not wanted.
- Typical dose: 40 µg bolus with a 2 min lockout.
- Side effect: respiratory depression – so high level of monitoring is required.

12.11 EPIDURAL ANALGESIA

Women offered epidural analgesia should be informed of the risks and benefits and the implications for their labour.

See Section 21.1 for the care of a woman who wishes to have epidural analgesia.

12.12 BLADDER CARE

Over-distension of the bladder could cause denervation and permanent damage to the bladder. Encourage the woman to empty her bladder at least every 3 hours, and document the volume passed. If she is unable to void urine after 4 hours, inform the doctor.

If an indwelling catheter is needed for any reason, use the smallest size possible, to reduce irritation of the urethra.

Vaginal delivery should not be conducted with a catheter still in place, since this could traumatise the urethra.

Fetal monitoring

13

A risk assessment is done on admission to the delivery suite. For low-risk women, the fetal heart may be auscultated intermittently using a fetal stethoscope (Pinard) or Doppler ultrasound (Sonicaid). See Sections 2.1 and 2.2 for a list of some conditions that exclude women from this group.

For at-risk women, a CTG is mandatory on admission. Continuous electronic monitoring is required in the following situations:

* Epidural sited
* Syntocinon infusion in progress
* Fresh meconium-stained amniotic fluid
* High-risk pregnancy (maternal or fetal problems)
* Maternal request
* Intermittent auscultation reveals decelerations
* Baseline fetal heart rate <110 or >160 beats/min
* Vaginal bleeding
* Maternal pyrexia

> ! Before commencing CTG or intermittent auscultation, palpate the maternal pulse simultaneously with auscultation to differentiate between maternal and fetal heart tones.

13.1 INTERMITTENT AUSCULTATION

Auscultate for 60 seconds, beginning immediately after the end of a contraction, every 15 minutes in the first stage of labour and every 5 minutes in the second stage.

13.2 ELECTRONIC FETAL MONITORING

Despite advances in digital recording and storage of CTGs, we still need paper copies.

* Check that the date and time clocks on the monitor are set correctly.
* Ensure that the paper speed is set to 1 cm/min.
* Label the paper with the woman's identifying details.
* If a good trace cannot be obtained using an abdominal transducer, then use a scalp electrode. If the signal is still poor, then the presence of fetal heart pulsation should be confirmed by an ultrasound scan.

DOI: 10.1201/9781315099897-16

FSE is contraindicated in:

- Women with HIV or hepatitis virus
- Fetal bleeding disorders (e.g. haemophilia)

13.3 SUSPICIOUS OR ABNORMAL TRACE

If any fetal heart rate abnormality is identified then monitoring should be continuous and, where necessary, an FSE should be applied. The coordinating midwife should be informed; if she/he is not happy then the doctor on call should be asked to review.

Any midwife or doctor reviewing a trace should document on both the trace and the case notes, stating their findings and plan.

When describing and acting on a CTG, the following features should be documented:

- Frequency and strength of uterine contractions
- Baseline fetal heart rate
- Variability
- Presence or absence of accelerations
- Presence or absence of decelerations
- Overall assessment and plan, taking into account any background risk

Every woman in labour having electronic fetal monitoring should have the trace reviewed at least every hour using the following classification (more frequently if there are concerns).

13.4 CLASSIFICATION OF CARDIOTOCOGRAPH (TABLE 13.1)

- **Normal:** all features of the cardiograph are normal.
- **Suspicious:** one feature is non-reassuring *and* two features are reassuring.
- **Pathological:** two features are non-reassuring, or there is at least one abnormal feature.

13.5 MANAGEMENT OF SUSPICIOUS OR PATHOLOGICAL CARDIOTOCOGRAPH

- The patient should be in the left lateral position.
- Inform the registrar.
- Check maternal pulse and temperature.
- Exclude hypotension; give crystalloid infusion if appropriate.

TABLE 13.1   Classification of Cardiotocograph

CLASSIFICATION	BASELINE (BEATS/MIN)	VARIABILITY	DECELERATION
Reassuring	110–160	5–25	None or Early Variable decelerations with no concerning characteristics* for less than 90 minutes
Non-reassuring	100–109, 161–180	<5 for 30–50 min	Early deceleration Variable decelerations with no concerning characteristics* for 90 minutes or more Variable decelerations with any concerning characteristics* in up to 50% of contractions for 30 minutes or more Variable decelerations with any concerning characteristics* in over 50% of contractions for less than 30 minutes Late decelerations in over 50% of contractions for less than 30 minutes, with no maternal or fetal clinical risk factors such as vaginal bleeding or significant meconium
Abnormal	<100, >180	<5 for ≥50 min OR >25 for more than 25 minutes OR Sinusoidal	Variable decelerations with any concerning characteristics* in over 50% of contractions for 30 minutes (or less if any maternal or fetal clinical risk factors [see above]) OR Late decelerations for 30 minutes (or less if any maternal or fetal clinical risk factors) OR Acute bradycardia, or a single prolonged deceleration lasting 3 minutes or more

- Exclude hypercontractility; stop Syntocinon infusion.
- Exclude cord prolapse (vaginal examination), placental abruption, uterine rupture.
- Review clinical situation for any other possible cause of abnormal CTG.
- Offer digital fetal scalp stimulation.
- If the trace is pathological or persistently suspicious, then FBS is indicated (see Chapter 14).
- Do not give oxygen to the mother, since it may be harmful to the hypoxic baby.

The presence of fetal heart rate accelerations, even with reduced baseline variability, is generally a sign that the baby is healthy.

If present, the following characteristics of variable decelerations are concerning:

- Lasting more than 60 seconds
- Reduced baseline variability within the deceleration
- Failure to return to baseline
- Biphasic (W) shape
- No shouldering

13.6 MANAGEMENT OF FETAL TACHYCARDIA

Ask the following questions:

- Is there an obvious explanation?
- How severe is the tachycardia?
- Are there other complications (decelerations, loss of variability) on the CTG?
- Is delivery imminent?

Take the following action:

- Check maternal pulse and temperature.
- Correct dehydration.
- If the fetal heart rate is 160–180 beats/min and the trace is uncomplicated, then no intervention is required.
- If the tachycardia is persistent and >180 beats/min, then do FBS. If FBS is not feasible, then discuss with the consultant and proceed to CS.

13.7 NOTE

In cases of fetal sepsis, there could be tachycardia with normal fetal scalp blood pH. Bear this in mind where there has been prolonged rupture of fetal membranes.

13.8 MANAGEMENT OF FETAL BRADYCARDIA

Prolonged deceleration for ≥3 minutes
   Assess the following:

- Depth of bradycardia
- Duration of bradycardia
- Signs of recovery (rapid or slow?)
- Variability
- Nature of the trace prior to bradycardia
- If in second stage, is delivery imminent?

Take the following action:

- Adopt left lateral tilt
- Turn off Syntocinon infusion
- Check and record maternal pulse
- Check BP

- If the woman is hypotensive or has just had an epidural, give a rapid infusion of IV fluid. (*Note*: following an epidural, a drop in fetal heart rate may occur even with a normal BP.)
- Perform a vaginal examination to exclude cord prolapse and to assess cervix and descent
- If there is vaginal bleeding, then consider the possibility of placental abruption or uterine rupture
- If there is no recovery by 6 minutes, prepare for operative delivery (CS or instrumental)
- If recovery occurs, reassess clinical situation

Scalp pH should not be performed for prolonged bradycardia.

> ! If there is bradycardia lasting up to 9 minutes, then proceed straight to CS (or instrumental delivery if feasible).

13.9 SCHEDULE

- **1–5 minutes**: call for help. Review as outlined earlier.
- **6 minutes**: expect recovery towards baseline. If there is no recovery, then prepare for operative delivery.
- **9 minutes**: if there is no recovery, transfer to theatre (or effect instrumental delivery if feasible).
- **15 minutes**: baby delivered.

13.10 REDUCED VARIABILITY (2–5 BEATS/MIN)

- This may reflect fetal sleep.
- Has the mother had a narcotic drug or sedation?
- If it lasts longer than 40 minutes, then do FBS (or discuss with consultant if FBS is not feasible).

Absent variability (<2 beats/min) calls for immediate intervention. Offer digital scalp stimulation.

When interpreting a complicated CTG, pay particular attention to the variability.

A more accurate picture of variability is obtained from a scalp electrode than from an abdominal transducer. The latter tends to overestimate variability.

13.11 LATE DECELERATION

Take the following action:

- Adopt left lateral tilt
- Turn off Syntocinon infusion
- Check BP
- Perform a vaginal examination to exclude cord prolapse and to assess cervix and descent
- If the cervix is ≥3 cm dilated, then do FBS. If it is <3 cm dilated, then proceed to CS

Decelerations in the second stage of labour may be innocent or indicative of hypoxia.
Assess the following:

- Nature of trace in the first stage of labour
- Depth, duration and recovery of decelerations
- Variability

If these give cause for concern, then operative delivery is indicated (see also 'Contraindications to FBS' in Chapter 14).

Fetal scalp blood sampling

14

If the CTG is suggestive of fetal distress, then FBS from the scalp should always be undertaken before proceeding to CS, unless it is technically not possible to do so.

- Explain the procedure to the woman and obtain consent.
- The cervix must be at least 3 cm dilated and the presenting part should be no more than 2 cm above the plane of the ischial spines.
- The patient should be in the left lateral position or in the lithotomy position with a wedge.
- At least two samples should be taken on each occasion. After obtaining each sample, ensure haemostasis by applying pressure with a swab on the stab site.
- Inform the patient of the result and plan.

14.1 CONTRAINDICATIONS TO FBS

- Prolonged (>10 minutes) fetal bradycardia
- Pathological CTG associated with APH, suspected chorioamnionitis or possible rupture of uterine scar
- Pregnancy <34 weeks
- Full cervical dilatation and presenting part below spines – **deliver the baby!**
- HIV-positive or hepatitis B-positive/C-positive mother; active herpes
- Fetal bleeding disorder (e.g. haemophilia)

14.2 INTERPRETATION OF PH RESULT

14.2.1 Normal values

- pH >7.25
- pO_2 >2.6 kPa (>20 mmHg) (note that pO_2 is not of value in assessing risk to the baby)
- pCO_2 <8 kPa (<50 mmHg)
- Base excess >8 mmol/L

Results should be interpreted in the context of clinical features, rate of progress in labour and previous pH reading:

- **≥7.25:** normal; may need repeating if CTG abnormality persists. If the FBS result is stable after the second test then, provided that there are no additional abnormalities on the trace, a third test may be deferred.
- **≤7.20:** acidosis; delivery indicated.
- **7.21–7.24:** repeat within 30 minutes or consider delivery if there has been a rapid fall since the last sample.

If two neat samples were obtained, management should be based on the lower pH. If no good sample was obtained, FBS should be repeated – do not derive false reassurance from an inadequate sample.

14.3 SCALP BLOOD LACTATE

This is an alternative to pH measurement and is done using commercially available test strips. Anaerobic metabolism produces lactate, so levels of this metabolite are a measure of tissue hypoxia. Optimal cut off level: 4.8 mmol/L.

Measurement of lactate in fetal scalp blood requires a smaller volume of blood and its predictive value for fetal acidosis is similar to that of pH measurement. It is not in widespread use in the UK.

14.4 DOCUMENTATION

- Obtain verbal consent
- The pH meter printout, labelled and dated, should be secured with sticky tape in the case notes
- Document the plan of management following blood sampling

14.5 FBS AT FULL CERVICAL DILATATION

If the cervix is fully dilated and the presenting part is below the plane of the ischial spines, then the woman should be offered instrumental delivery.

If the presenting part is still high, FBS may be performed. A normal result allows time for descent of the presenting part, thus allowing a normal delivery or increasing the chances of a successful instrumental delivery.

! If FBS has been performed, then cord-blood sampling should be performed at delivery.

Augmentation of labour

15

If labour is slow, then consider the following possible causes:

- Prolonged latent phase of labour (safe to augment)
- Inefficient uterine activity (generally safe to augment)
- Obstructed labour (dangerous to augment)

15.1 ARTIFICIAL RUPTURE OF FETAL MEMBRANES (ARM)

'The older doctrine of the sanctity of the membranes was more or less built in with the bricks in my obstetrical philosophy. No labour is so pleasing and satisfactory to mother and child as when intact membranes are maintained right up to full dilatation at which point a gush of clear, clean liquor amnii flushes out the genital tract, followed, not so many minutes later, by the delivery of a clean, healthy, screaming baby. This is Nature at her best and I never cease to marvel at such normality'.

Donald I. *Practical Obstetric Problems*, 5th edn.
London: Lloyd-Luke, 1979:566

ARM should not be performed routinely, but it may be used to accelerate labour if progress is slow (<1 cm/h). It should be discussed with the woman before the vaginal examination is performed.

The rate of progress must be considered in the context of the mother's circumstances. A rate of 1 cm/h in a woman who is having strong uterine contractions and who is in severe distress is more worrying than a rate of 0.5 cm/h in a woman who is comfortable and mobile.

The midwife may rupture the membranes artificially (for induction or augmentation of labour) if the following criteria are met and the mother consents:

- The head is engaged
- The vertex is presenting
- Cord presentation has been excluded

Contraindications to ARM are:

- Abnormal lie
- Cord presentation
- Placenta praevia

After ARM, check for cord prolapse and meconium staining of amniotic fluid. Document the fetal heart rate.

DOI: 10.1201/9781315099897-18

15.2 AUGMENTATION WITH SYNTOCINON

Syntocinon (oxytocin) may be prescribed to accelerate labour, provided that the following conditions are met:

- Presentation is cephalic
- Membranes have ruptured
- Amniotic fluid is clear

Syntocinon infusion should not be started until 6 hours have elapsed since administration of prostaglandin (risk of uterine tachysystole).

Syntocinon should not be used in secondary arrest (after 5 cm dilatation) until obstructed labour has been excluded by vaginal examination. Particular care should be taken in multiparous women.

The use of Syntocinon in the following circumstances requires the explicit approval of the consultant:

- Multiple pregnancy
- Malpresentation
- Previous CS or other uterine scar
- Grandmultiparity

If augmentation of labour is indicated then the midwife, per patient group direction, may commence an IV infusion of Syntocinon:

- If maternal and fetal wellbeing are normal
- Following discussion with obstetrician on call
- With documentation in labour records

When labour is augmented with Syntocinon, a vaginal examination should be performed 4 hours after commencing the infusion. If there is less than 2 cm progress after 4 hours of Syntocinon, then CS should be considered.

15.3 SYNTOCINON INFUSION

Mix 10 units of Syntocinon in 500 mL Hartmann's solution. Commence infusion at 2 milliunits/min (i.e. 6 mL/h). Increase every 30 minutes until strong, regular uterine contractions – three in 10 minutes – are obtained.

- A syringe driver or infusion pump must be used.
- Do not exceed 32 milliunits/min (i.e. 96 mL/h); see Table 15.1.
- Do not infuse through the same line as blood, plasma or insulin.
- The syringe must be labelled, with the dose of drug and signatures of responsible staff on the label.
- All women for whom labour is being augmented with Syntocinon should have continuous electronic fetal monitoring.

15.4 SECOND STAGE OF LABOUR

Syntocinon infusion may be given to augment uterine contractions in the second stage of labour, providing that obstructed labour has been excluded by abdominal and vaginal examination.

Mix 10 units of Syntocinon in 500 mL Hartmann's solution. Commence infusion at 2 milliunits/min (i.e. 6 mL/h). Increase every 15 minutes until strong, regular uterine contractions – three in 10 minutes – are obtained.

15.5 UTERINE HYPERSTIMULATION

- More than five contractions per 10-minute interval for at least 20 minutes (uterine tachysystole), or each uterine contraction lasting up to 2 minutes or increased baseline uterine tone (uterine hypertonus).
- Suspicious or pathological CTG.

15.6 MANAGEMENT

- Discontinue Syntocinon infusion
- Lay the woman on her left side
- Institute a rapid infusion of 1000 mL 0.9% saline
- In extreme cases, consider tocolysis with terbutaline 0.25 mg SC. *Note*: This is an off-licence use of terbutaline
- It may be necessary to deliver the baby – is the CTG back to normal?

TABLE 15.1   Regimen for Syntocinon Infusion

TIME AFTER STARTING (MIN)	RATE (MILLIUNITS/MIN)	RATE (ML/H)
0	2	6
30	4	12
60	8	24
90	12	36
120	16	48
150	20	60
180	24	72
210	28	84
240	32	96

Cord-blood sampling

16

Blood should be obtained for acid–base status from an isolated segment of umbilical cord following delivery of any potentially acidotic fetus, including:

- Intrapartum CTG
- Cases where fetal scalp blood has been sampled
- Instrumental vaginal delivery
- Preterm delivery
- Breech vaginal delivery
- IUGR
- Placental abruption
- Cord prolapse
- Baby born with a low Apgar score
- Fetal abnormality

A quality control check must be made on the analyser as directed by the manufacturer (see the handbook accompanying the machine).

A 10 cm segment of cord is clamped immediately after delivery of the baby.

Samples of cord artery and vein are obtained with pre-heparinized syringes. The arterial sample is more difficult to obtain, but this is the sample that is representative of the baby's acid–base balance. Unless both arterial and venous samples are obtained, it cannot be established that the umbilical artery has been sampled.

The segment of cord (or the sample in the pre-heparinized syringe) may be left at room temperature for up to 30 minutes (or in ice for up to 1 hour) before analysis.

Inform the duty paediatrician if the arterial pH <7.05 or if the venous pH <7.20.

> **!** Beware – with some analysers, the quality control printout could be mistaken for the actual specimen result.

DOI: 10.1201/9781315099897-19

Epidural analgesia in labour

17

Epidural analgesia in labour requires a resident anaesthetist and continuous care and monitoring of the mother and fetus by a suitably trained midwife. If either is unavailable, then epidural analgesia should not be instituted. Patient information about epidurals and other forms of pain relief should be available.

The woman should be informed that epidural analgesia is associated with a longer second stage of labour and an increased chance of vaginal instrumental birth but is not associated with long-term back-ache or with a longer first stage of labour or an increased chance of caesarean birth. If the epidural solution contains opioids, the mother should be informed of the risk of short-term respiratory depression and drowsiness in the baby.

17.1 INDICATIONS FOR EPIDURAL ANALGESIA

- Maternal request
- Occipito-posterior position
- Induced/accelerated labour
- Prolonged labour
- Multiple pregnancy
- Breech presentation
- Pre-eclampsia (see later)
- Premature birth/high-risk fetus
- Maternal medical problems (e.g. diabetes, asthma and certain cardiac problems)

17.2 CONTRAINDICATIONS TO EPIDURAL ANALGESIA

- Maternal refusal
- Coagulopathy (see later)
- Shock/uncorrected hypovolaemia
- Inadequate staffing
- Septicaemia
- Local infection
- Raised intracranial pressure
- Allergy to amide local anaesthetics (rare)

DOI: 10.1201/9781315099897-20

17.3 COAGULOPATHY

The risks and benefits of epidural analgesia/anaesthesia need to be assessed in each case. It is not possible to lay down absolute criteria. A regional block is usually given if the platelet count is above 100×10^9/L, but epidural analgesia may be withheld if the count is higher than this but falling rapidly. A coagulation profile must be done if the platelet count is $<100 \times 10^9$/L, and a senior anaesthetist must be involved.

A platelet count should be done in the case of pre-eclampsia and where there has previously been a low count.

In addition, PT, APTT and FDPs should be checked in the following cases:

- Severe pre-eclampsia (including HELLP)
- Intrauterine death
- Placental abruption

17.4 THERAPEUTIC/PROPHYLACTIC ANTICOAGULATION

Some women will have had LMWH – usually dalteparin (Fragmin) – for prophylaxis or treatment of thrombosis. This is not an absolute contraindication to regional block.

Peak anti-Xa activity (see Glossary) is reached about 3 hours after a subcutaneous injection of LMWH, but 50% of peak levels are still present at 12 hours. Spinal/epidural should be inserted at least 12 hours after a prophylactic dose and 24 hours after a therapeutic dose. Patients on any anticoagulant should have PT and APTT checked before placing an epidural/spinal but note that these are unlikely to be affected by LMWH.

17.5 SETTING UP

Exact equipment requirements vary between anaesthetists. The following are usually required:

- IV cannula (minimum 16G, i.e. grey Venflon) with a 1000 mL bag of Hartmann's solution connected via a blood-giving set
- Epidural trolley, fully stocked (the stock list is on the trolley)
- Resuscitation equipment, including oxygen and suction
- Patient's records and an epidural chart
- BP and fetal heart monitoring equipment
- Tilting bed
- Wedge

The anaesthetist will want to know:

- Parity
- Whether there has been a previous epidural

- Stage and progress of labour
- Other analgesia used. *Women who have had intramuscular pethidine should not receive an epidural containing opiate for 4 hours post the injection.*
- Significant obstetric and medical problems
- Maternal BP and vaginal examination findings

17.6 PROCEDURE

- The procedure is explained by the anaesthetist. Verbal consent is obtained and documented.
- Ask the woman to empty her bladder.
- A preload of IV fluid may be given but is not routinely required before establishing low-dose epidural analgesia and combined spinal–epidural analgesia. The drip must be able to flow freely if needed.
- The woman should be either on her side or sitting on the side of the bed and leaning over a table.
- An appropriate area of the back (L2–3 or L3–4) should be cleaned with chlorhexidine spray.
- The midwife should support the mother during the procedure, particularly with regard to maintaining good position.
- After catheter insertion, a test dose of local anaesthetic is given to exclude placement in the cerebrospinal fluid or a vein.
- BP and pulse rate should be checked every 5 minutes for a further 15–20 minutes, during which time the mother should not be left unattended.

17.7 METHOD OF ADMINISTRATION

When the epidural catheter has been inserted, continuous analgesia can be administered by one of the following means:

- Infusion
- Boluses (top-ups)
- Controlled epidural analgesia
- Spinal epidural

17.8 EPIDURAL INFUSION

Continuous infusion reduces, but does not eliminate, the need for bolus injections. Often at least one top-up is required. There are two reasons for this:

- Epidural drug requirements tend to increase as labour progresses.
- Infusion rates sufficient to eliminate the need for top-ups often cause excessive blocks and are therefore best avoided.

TABLE 17.1   Adjustments to Infusion Rate When There Is a Problem

FINDING	ACTION
Mother in pain	Administer top-up and increase rate by 2 mL/h
Epigastric cold/pinch	Reduce rate by 2 mL/h
Sensation abnormal	Recheck in 30 min
Excessive motor block	Reduce rate by 2 mL/h
	Recheck in 30 min

The anaesthetist will prescribe a low-dose anaesthetic agent (e.g. 10–20 mL of 0.1% bupivacaine with 1–2 micrograms/mL fentanyl) and the infusion rate. When indicated, the infusion rate should be adjusted as outlined in Table 17.1.

High concentrations of local anaesthetic solutions (≥0.25% of bupivacaine or equivalent) should not be used routinely for either establishing or maintaining epidural analgesia.

The following observations are required hourly:

- Volume infused
- Infusion rate
- Presence or absence of excessive motor block (inability to bend both knees)
- Block height (test for cold sensation or pinch in the epigastrium; sensation should be normal here)

Inform the anaesthetist if:

- Pain does not respond to a top-up after 20 minutes.
- Abnormal epigastric sensation persists 30 minutes after reducing the infusion rate.
- Excessive motor block persists 30 minutes after reducing the infusion rate.

17.9 EPIDURAL TOP-UP

A trained midwife may give top-ups of anaesthetic in doses prescribed by the anaesthetist. The anaesthetist must be available within 5 minutes if there are problems. Typical dose: 15 mL of 0.1% bupivacaine with 2 µg/mL fentanyl, given every hour.

17.10 PROTOCOL FOR TOP-UPS

- A top-up is indicated if the mother is in pain and feels that her analgesia is inadequate.
- Check epidural prescription (**do not rely on oral instructions**).
- Check maternal pulse and BP, motor block and block height. Contact the anaesthetist if there are any adverse findings.
- Check bladder fullness and empty as necessary.

- Draw up the prescribed dose of anaesthetic agent. **This must be checked with a second midwife**.
- Do not administer epidural drugs during a contraction.
- The mother should be in a sitting or full lateral position.
- Administer the drug in a divided dose.
- The initial fraction must be given *slowly*. Over the next 5 minutes, observe/ask about any sudden increase in motor block, dizziness, tingling in the face and tinnitus.
- At 5 minutes, check maternal pulse and BP. **The upper arm will under-read BP if the patient is in a lateral position**. If dizziness, tingling or another symptom is observed or if the systolic BP falls below 90 mmHg (or by >30 mmHg), then omit the remaining fraction and call the anaesthetist. Otherwise, administer the remaining dose and continue observing for these symptoms or hypotension.
- Check BP every 5 minutes for a further 15–20 minutes. The woman must not be left unattended during this time.

! If the top-up is ineffective after 20 minutes, call the anaesthetist.

If hypotension occurs at any stage, treat as outlined under 'Hypotension' on Section 17.13.1 and call the anaesthetist.

17.11 GENERAL CARE OF THE WOMAN WITH AN EPIDURAL

The woman should be looked after by a dedicated and suitably trained midwife. The anaesthetist remains responsible for the regional block and should attend regularly, not just when called by the midwife.

If the midwife has any concerns about the epidural (see 'Complications' later) then the anaesthetist should be contacted.

The woman should be encouraged to move and adopt whatever upright positions she finds comfortable throughout labour. **She should never be supine**. If she is on her back, then a wedge must be always under the right buttock, even during vaginal examination. At other times, the sitting position is preferred. If the woman wishes to lie down, then the full lateral position is acceptable.

- Hourly position changes (to avoid pressure-related problems) should be continued until the epidural has worn off completely and should be recorded on the appropriate chart.
- Maternal BP should be checked every 30 minutes.
- There should be continuous fetal heart monitoring (note that CTG abnormalities may occur up to 1 hour after an epidural).
- Temperature should be checked every 4 hours.
- Encourage bladder emptying every 2 hours and before top-ups. Palpate regularly to detect urinary retention. Record urine output.
- Perform vaginal examination as indicated (with wedge in place).

17.12 IN THE SECOND STAGE OF LABOUR

- Breakthrough pain may occur. A top-up should be offered. This should be given in the sitting position to block the sacral root.
- The epidural infusion should not be stopped. If the woman is totally unaware of her contractions (which is not common in practice), then she should be encouraged to push when contractions are palpated. The prescribed infusion rate may be reduced by 2 mL/h in these circumstances. There is insufficient evidence to suggest that stopping an epidural late in labour lowers the risk of instrumental delivery or other unwanted outcomes.
- In the second stage of labour, unless the woman has an urge to push or the baby's head is visible, pushing should be delayed for at least 1 hour – longer if the woman wishes – after which pushing during contractions should be actively encouraged.
- Perineal infiltration may still be required before episiotomy.

17.13 COMPLICATIONS OF EPIDURAL ANALGESIA

- Inadequate analgesia

This may occur at some stage in up to 20% of epidurals.
    Give a top-up as detailed earlier and call the anaesthetist if this is ineffective after 20 minutes.

- Hypotension

17.13.1 Prevention of hypotension

- Make the appropriate checks before giving a bolus.
- The woman should always avoid the supine position.
- Correct any pre-existing hypovolaemia.

If the systolic BP falls below 90 mmHg (on the lower arm if the woman is in the lateral position):

- Turn the woman to the full lateral position. If this is ineffective, then:
- Fully open the drip and give 500 mL compound sodium lactate (Hartmann's solution).
- Give oxygen by facemask (minimum 10 L flow with wall oxygen).
- Call the anaesthetist.
- Have ready a box of ephedrine or phenylephrine, water for dilution and a 10 mL syringe. Administer this if the systolic blood pressure falls to less than 80 mmHg.

17.14 DURAL TAP

- This occurs when the epidural needle or catheter accidentally penetrates the dura, usually resulting in a leak of cerebrospinal fluid.

- Immediate management varies between cases. The anaesthetist will leave specific instructions.
- Any further bolus doses of local anaesthetic must be administered by the anaesthetist.
- **There is no evidence to support elective instrumental delivery.**
- Inform the woman of the puncture.
- Inform the anaesthetist if the woman develops a headache.

17.15 LOCAL ANAESTHETIC TOXICITY (IV INJECTION)

Suspect this if the epidural catheter is blood-stained and the epidural not effective. Features include metallic taste, tinnitus, tingling in the face, dizziness, confusion, slurred speech, arrhythmia, seizures, loss of consciousness and cardiovascular collapse. If the woman has any of these during a bolus, stop the injection and call the anaesthetist. Turn the woman to the lateral position, give oxygen and check her vital signs.

The epidural catheter should always be aspirated gently before giving any injection of local anaesthetic solution, to exclude intravascular position.

17.16 TOTAL SPINAL

This occurs when the catheter is placed intrathecally. *The epidural catheter should always be aspirated gently before giving any injection of local anaesthetic solution.*

The features are rapid onset of analgesia and a dense motor block, followed by nausea and vomiting, pallor and sweating, possibly leading to loss of consciousness and apnoea (cessation of breathing).

BP will be very low. Maternal heart rate may be high or low. The fetal heart will almost certainly deteriorate.

Initial treatment is as for hypotension:

- Place the woman in the full lateral position.
- Open the drip fully.
- Give oxygen by mask (this may need the support of breathing; check breathing and commence basic life support if needed).
- Call the anaesthetist.
- Have ephedrine/phenylephrine, atropine and a cardiac arrest trolley ready in the room.
- Alert the obstetrician – emergency delivery likely to be needed.

17.17 DENSE MOTOR BLOCK

The woman should not mobilize until motor block has worn off. The block has worn off when the woman is able to straight-leg raise, bring her knees up to her chest, and push hard against resistance with both feet, without difficulty in both lower limbs.

- **Change her position hourly** to prevent pressure-related problems. These should be continued until the motor block has worn off completely.

17.18 BLADDER DISTENSION

Regular voiding should be encouraged during labour, particularly before a bolus is given and until the epidural has worn off. Distension may be palpable and/or may cause breakthrough pain. In-and-out catheterization should be performed if the woman is unable to void spontaneously.

! Call the anaesthetist if any of the following occur:
- Inadequate anaesthesia
  - Hypotension
  - Headache following dural tap
  - Symptoms of local anaesthetic toxicity (see previous page)
  - Dense motor block
- Any other concern

17.19 DISCONTINUATION OF EPIDURAL

- After delivery, remove the catheter with a gentle, steady pull, ideally with the woman in the same position as during insertion. The tip of the catheter should be checked for completeness and a record made.
- Before removing the catheter, always check whether LMWH was given. If LMWH was given, at least 12 hours must elapse before the catheter is removed.
- The woman should not be allowed to mobilize until she is able to flex both hips and knees against resistance. She should be accompanied when she first walks.

Management of the second stage of labour

18

The second stage of labour comprises:

a. **passive second stage:** the cervix is fully dilated but there are no involuntary expulsive contractions
b. **active second stage:** the cervix is fully dilated, there are involuntary expulsive contractions and the baby is visible

Once the second stage has been diagnosed, the woman should not be left without a midwife in attendance. Essential elements of care commenced in the first stage of labour – such as psychological support and hydration – should be continued in the second stage.

The woman should be encouraged to give birth in the position that she finds most comfortable. The recumbent position tends to lengthen labour, to reduce the incidence of spontaneous birth and to increase the incidence of abnormal fetal heart rate patterns.

Regardless of whether it is a normal delivery or an instrumental delivery, only the accoucheur and no more than one assistant should be at the lower end of the woman's body.

Fetal heart rate should be recorded at least after every second contraction. BP should be recorded half-hourly if normal, but every 15 minutes in hypertensive women.

! Always be certain that the cervix is fully dilated.

18.1 DURATION

There is no evidence to suggest that the imposition of an upper time limit for the duration of the second stage improves the outcome for mother or baby. More important than the time factor are evidence of progressive descent and maternal and fetal wellbeing.

18.2 PASSIVE PHASE

Labour that is progressing normally may be in the passive stage for 1 hour. In a woman who has not had epidural analgesia, if the vertex is not visible within the hour, then a vaginal examination should be performed.

DOI: 10.1201/9781315099897-21

18.3 ACTIVE PHASE

The doctor should be informed if the baby has not been delivered after 2 hours of pushing in a nullipara or after 1 hour in a multipara.

18.4 IMMEDIATE VERSUS DELAYED PUSHING

A nulliparous woman with epidural analgesia may start pushing within an hour of full cervical dilatation (immediate pushing) or after up to 2 hours in the passive phase (delayed pushing). A meta-analysis of seven random-allocation trials showed that delayed pushing (passive descent) was associated with an increased chance of spontaneous vaginal births, a decreased risk of instrumental delivery and a shorter pushing time.

Encourage active pushing when:

- The woman has a desire to push, and the vertex is visible on gently parting the labia.
- 1 hour has elapsed since full dilatation was confirmed, and the presenting part is below the plane of the ischial spines.

Observations and assessment in second stage:

- Take BP and pulse hourly.
- Take temperature 4-hourly (continued from first stage).
- Document frequency of contractions at least half-hourly.
- Empty the bladder.
- Perform a vaginal examination after 60 minutes of pushing or where there is concern (e.g. cord prolapse).
- Measure fetal heart rate. If using intermittent auscultation, do this every 5 minutes.

Steady progress should be made in the active stage. Keep the coordinating midwife informed. Progress must be assessed by abdominal as well as vaginal examination.

18.5 DELAYED SECOND STAGE

Inform the doctor if:

- After 1 hour in the passive phase, the presenting part is not visible.
- A nulliparous woman is undelivered after 2 hours of active pushing.
- A multiparous woman is undelivered after 1 hour of active pushing.

18.6 MANAGEMENT OF DELAYED SECOND STAGE

- Exclude disproportion. Excessive caput and moulding are indicative of obstruction.
- If contractions are inadequate and there are no contraindications, commence Syntocinon (oxytocin) infusion. Contraindications include disproportion, abnormal CTG and possible rupture of scar.
- Evaluate for instrumental delivery.

A SITUATION TO BE AVOIDED:

'In the second stage it is common to see assistants crowding at the lower end of the woman's body, anxiously watching her vulva as if waiting for luggage to appear in an airport carousel.'

Sheila Kitzinger. Birth and violence against women – generating hypotheses from women's accounts of unhappiness after childbirth. In: Roberts H, ed. *Women's Health Matters*. London: Routledge, 1992:Chap 4

18.7 CALLING THE PAEDIATRICIAN

In some cases, it will be necessary to call the paediatrician in the second stage of labour, when delivery is imminent – see Chapter 19. It is advisable to document the time when this call is made.

Criteria for paediatric attendance at delivery

19

If any of the following are noted, a paediatrician should be called to attend the delivery:

- Fetal distress
- Abnormal presentation
- Prolapsed cord
- APH
- Meconium-stained amniotic fluid
- Forceps/vacuum-assisted delivery (except lift-out procedures, where there is no fetal distress)
- CS if performed under general anaesthesia or if there is a fetal indication (e.g. IUGR)
- Severe pre-eclampsia
- Drug abuse/addiction by mother
- Diabetes mellitus
- Multiple pregnancy
- Breech vaginal delivery
- Preterm delivery (<36 weeks)
- Rh isoimmunization
- Fetal hydrops
- Polyhydramnios
- Congenital abnormalities
- Anticipated shoulder dystocia
- Concern of attending midwife/obstetrician

The gestational age and reason for requesting neonatology team attendance should be stated when the team is bleeped.

In the case of prolonged rupture of membranes (>24 hours), ear and umbilical swabs should be obtained from the baby and the paediatrician should be informed.

> ! The midwife or obstetrician should use their clinical judgement to determine whether to call the first on-call or second on-call paediatrician, depending on the degree of risk.

DOI: 10.1201/9781315099897-22

Management of the third stage of labour

20

Active management of the third stage of labour significantly reduces the risk of PPH, regardless of the posture of the mother or the experience of the midwife, but there is a slight increase in the incidence of nausea and vomiting.

Active management is the recommended practice unless the mother makes an informed choice to have physiological management. The mother's choice should be documented clearly on her birth plan and labour record.

A combination of active and physiological management is unacceptable.

Physiological management is contraindicated in the following circumstances:

- Operative delivery
- Induced or augmented labour
- Polyhydramnios
- Previous PPH
- Epidural analgesia
- Diabetes mellitus
- Prolonged labour
- Multiple pregnancy
- APH
- Anticoagulant therapy
- Anaemia
- Grandmultiparity

20.1 ACTIVE MANAGEMENT

1. Give an oxytocic drug with delivery of the anterior shoulder. IM Syntometrine (ergometrine with oxytocin) 1 mL to the upper thigh muscle is the drug of choice unless contraindicated, in which case give IM Syntocinon (oxytocin) 10 IU.
   Contraindications to Syntometrine:

   - Hypertension, pre-eclampsia
   - Severe cardiac disease
   - Pulmonary oedema
   - Hepatic or renal impairment

DOI: 10.1201/9781315099897-23

The World Health Organization (WHO) recommends the use of carbetocin, an analogue of oxytocin, in low- and middle-income countries, as it is heat-stable and does not require cold chain for storage and transport (single intravenous dose of 100 mcg, slowly over 1 minute.

2. Clamp the cord 1–3 minutes after birth.
3. Deliver the placenta and membranes by controlled cord traction with the next uterine contraction.

20.2 IF THE PLACENTA IS NOT DELIVERED WITHIN 30 MINUTES, REFER TO THE OBSTETRICIAN

20.3 PHYSIOLOGICAL MANAGEMENT

- Do not give any oxytocic drug.
- Leave the cord to pulsate; do not clamp or cut.
- Adopt careful watching and waiting. Do not apply any cord traction.
- Encourage breastfeeding.
- Observe for signs of separation: lengthening of cord, gush of blood or rise of the uterine fundus.
- Encourage maternal effort aided by gravity.
- **If the placenta is not delivered within 1 hour (earlier if there is concern regarding blood loss or maternal condition), then refer to the obstetrician.**

Immediate postpartum care
21

It is advisable for the mother and baby to remain in the midwife's care, on the delivery suite, for 1 hour after delivery. If there are any deviations from normal wellbeing of the mother or the infant, then the obstetrician or paediatrician must agree transfer to the postnatal ward.

The drug chart should be checked before transfer to the ward to ensure that analgesics, antibiotics, thromboembolism prophylaxis and other medication have been prescribed as required.

21.1 CARE OF THE MOTHER

The mother's general wellbeing, pulse, BP and temperature should be recorded. Assessment of uterine retraction and vaginal blood loss should also be documented. The mother should be offered a bed bath or shower, as well as light refreshment, and made comfortable before arrangements for her transfer to the postnatal ward.

If an epidural catheter is in place, it should be removed before the mother leaves the delivery suite. The tip of the catheter should be checked for completeness and a record made.

21.2 BLADDER CARE

Over-distension of the bladder could cause denervation and permanent damage to the bladder. Ensure that the woman has voided urine prior to leaving the delivery suite and document the time and volume of the first void. If she has not voided, inform the staff on the postnatal ward. If a woman has not voided urine 6 hours post-delivery, a catheter should be introduced. A bladder scan could also be used to determine whether the bladder is full.

It can take 8 hours for the bladder to regain sensation after epidural analgesia. Women who have had spinal or epidural analgesia for operative delivery should have an indwelling catheter for at least 12 hours.

Women with any of the following conditions are at risk of acute urinary retention:

- Difficult vaginal birth with perineal/vulval trauma and suturing
- Prolonged labour
- Epidural analgesia during labour
- Vaginal or postoperative abdominal pain
- History of voiding problems

DOI: 10.1201/9781315099897-24

21.3 CARE OF THE BABY

See Chapter 22.

21.4 THE PLACENTA

The placenta should be examined and the findings documented. The following checks should be performed:

- What is the overall appearance: normal/gritty/small or large?
- Are the cotyledons complete?
- Are the membranes complete or ragged?
- Is the insertion of the cord vessels normal or abnormal?

In some cases – such as twin births, stillbirths and other adverse outcomes – it may be advisable to send the placenta for histopathological examination.

21.5 DOCUMENTATION

The midwife is responsible for seeing that all observations are made and recorded before transfer to the postnatal ward:

- Case records (mother and baby)
- Birth register
- Maternity information system (computer)

Any deviations from normal should be reported to the obstetrician on duty.

Care of the newborn 22

> ! For most infants, the needs after delivery are a warm welcome, clear airway and vigilance.

No benefits have been demonstrated for the routine suctioning of the newborn's oral and nasal passages. However, if there has been any indication of meconium-stained amniotic fluid, then the paediatrician should be called to delivery and the airways cleared under direct vision. The oropharynx should always be cleared before the nasal passages. The aspiration of meconium from the nose and mouth of the unborn baby while the head is still on the perineum is not recommended.

22.1 SKIN-TO-SKIN CONTACT

The benefits of skin-to-skin contact are:

- Maintenance of the baby's body temperature
- More successful breastfeeding

The mother, regardless of whether she intends to breastfeed or formula-feed, should be encouraged to have skin-to-skin contact with the infant immediately following delivery. If the mother is not able to do this, the partner may be able to offer skin-to-skin contact.

Skin-to-skin contact may be delayed where there are concerns about the wellbeing of the mother or baby, but it should not be delayed or interrupted by routine procedures such as weighing the baby.

For a baby requiring resuscitation, skin-to-skin contact should be established once the baby has been resuscitated.

The first feed is given once the baby shows signs of readiness (sucking, rooting and hand-to-mouth movements).

- Skin-to-skin contact (or its refusal) should be documented.

22.2 PREVENTION OF HYPOTHERMIA

Hypothermia is a core temperature of less than 35°C. Heat loss is more rapid, and consequences are more severe in immature babies.

DOI: 10.1201/9781315099897-25

The ideal delivery-suite environment for a baby is:

- Still air
- Temperature 34°C
- 100% relative humidity

Therefore:

- Optimize the temperature.
- Ensure that the room is not draughty.
- Dry the baby at birth and wrap in a dry towel.
- If resuscitation is required, use a Resuscitaire (i.e. place the baby under radiant heat).

22.3 VITAMIN K

Vitamin K prophylaxis at birth prevents bleeding due to vitamin K deficiency (formerly known as haemorrhagic disease of the newborn). Information regarding the use of vitamin K should be given to all mothers. Valid parental consent should be obtained and documented.

22.3.1 Routes of administration

- **Intramuscular**: vitamin K 1 mg IM. This is inexpensive and easy to administer. There was some concern about possible links with childhood cancer, but further studies found no link between vitamin K and cancer. Parenteral injection in premature babies is associated with an increased risk of kernicterus, so babies weighing less than 1500 g should receive the lower dose of 0.5 mg IM.
- **Oral**: Konakion MM Paediatric, 2 mg at birth and 2 mg within the next 7 days. For breastfed babies, a further 2 mg dose is given at 1 month; this dose is omitted in formula-fed babies because formula feeds contain vitamin K.

Standard practice is to use the injectable vitamin K preparation. Where parents opt for the oral preparation, refer to patient group direction.

If oral vitamin K has been chosen by a breastfeeding mother, then adequate arrangements should be made between the midwife, health visitor, GP and parents to ensure that the third dose is given at 1 month.

Vitamin K is indicated particularly in babies of women who have taken anticonvulsants (e.g. phenytoin) or oral anticoagulants in pregnancy.

22.4 IDENTIFICATION OF THE BABY

The delivering/supervising midwife is responsible for ensuring that the baby is wearing an identification band before leaving the labour ward.

- Attach an identifying band securely to each ankle of the baby. This should be done in the presence of the mother if possible. The baby's name and the mother's hospital number should be written clearly on each band.

22.5 BREASTFEEDING

This should be encouraged as soon as possible after delivery.

22.6 MANAGEMENT OF HYPOGLYCAEMIA

Hypoglycaemia is a blood glucose level <2.7 mmol/L.
   The following are associated with an increased risk of hypoglycaemia:

- Preterm birth
- Small for gestational age (below the third centile)
- Macrosomia
- Diabetic mother
- Hypothermia

Signs include cold, sweatiness, jitteriness, behaviour changes, floppiness, apnoea, cyanosis and pallor. Babies with any of these signs should have their blood glucose measured.
   Urgent action is required:

- Inform the paediatrician
- Give glucose as prescribed by the paediatrician. The baby may have to be transferred to the SCBU

22.7 PREVENTIVE CARE

Babies small for gestational age, and other babies at increased risk, should have:

- Feeding (within 2 hours of delivery)
- Feeding (3-hourly)
- Glucose checked (dipstick) before each feed in the first 48 hours

Meconium-stained amniotic fluid

23

23.1 RISK TO BABY

The baby is at risk of meconium aspiration syndrome. The risk is more significant when there is thick meconium.

23.2 NOTE

Amnioinfusion is not recommended for the management of meconium-stained amniotic fluid.

23.3 MECONIUM-STAINED FLUID IN LABOUR

- Inform the paediatrician
- Prepare Resuscitaire and endotracheal tubes
- Obtain a CTG

23.4 MECONIUM-STAINED FLUID AT VAGINAL DELIVERY

Do not suck the mouth and nostrils prior to birth of the shoulders and trunk. You can do so after birth, but only if the baby has thick meconium in the oropharynx. Aspiration of meconium from the nose and mouth of the unborn baby while the head is still on the perineum is not recommended.

If the baby is pink, vigorous and not in respiratory distress, then no further resuscitation is necessary.

If the baby is floppy at birth, then visualize the vocal cord (by laryngoscopy) and suck if necessary.

If no meconium is seen below the cord and the Apgar score at 5 minutes is greater than 8 and the baby is asymptomatic:

- Observe on the postnatal ward – respiration, feeding and finger-prick glucose.
- The paediatrician should review at 1–2 hours.
- The following observations should be recorded at 1 hour, 2 hours and then 2-hourly for 10 hours:

DOI: 10.1201/9781315099897-26

- General wellbeing
- Chest movements and nasal flare
- Skin colour, including perfusion by testing capillary refill
- Feeding
- Muscle tone
- Temperature
- Heart rate and respiration

Admit into SCBU for observation if:

- Meconium is seen below the cord
- There is respiratory distress
- The baby is still floppy at 5 minutes

If the mother has had pethidine in the last 4 hours, give naloxone to the baby and observe for 10 minutes. If the baby is still floppy, admit to SCBU.

Check cord blood gases.

23.5 MECONIUM-STAINED FLUID AT CAESAREAN SECTION

Transfer immediately to Resuscitaire. The principles are then the same as mentioned earlier.

Neonatal resuscitation

24

All midwives, obstetricians and paediatricians have a responsibility to achieve and maintain the skills needed for neonatal resuscitation.

A list of equipment and drugs is kept in the delivery rooms, obstetric theatre and on Resuscitaires.

All delivery rooms, obstetric theatres and Resuscitaires must be checked daily and before use.

All equipment and drugs used during resuscitation must be replaced as soon as possible.

Heaters should be turned on and warm towels should be readily available.

24.1 PRINCIPLES

At the onset of acute hypoxia, fetal breathing movements become more rapid. As oxygen levels continue to fall, regular breathing movements cease, since the centres responsible for controlling them are unable to function owing to lack of oxygen. The fetus enters a period known as **primary apnoea**. The heart rate falls but the BP is maintained.

If the hypoxia continues and the fetus is not delivered, gasping activity begins. As the gasps fail to aerate the lungs, they fade away. This is because increasing acidosis and hypoxia interfere with the ability of the heart muscle to function effectively. The gasps eventually cease and the fetus enters **secondary** or **terminal apnoea**.

Infants in primary apnoea will quickly recover if the airway is open and oxygenated blood is transported to the heart and lungs. If the infant is in terminal apnoea, he/she will not recover without intervention and may die despite receiving help. It is not possible to distinguish whether an infant who is not breathing at birth is in primary apnoea and about to gasp or has taken his/her last gasp in utero and is now in terminal apnoea.

> ! All infants born apnoeic must be presumed to be in terminal apnoea.

24.2 AVOID THERMAL STRESS

Keep the baby dry and warm: all infants must be dried thoroughly and wrapped in clean, warm towels. Cold stress increases metabolic acidosis.

DOI: 10.1201/9781315099897-27

24.2.1 The temperature of newborn infants should be maintained between 36.5°C and 37.5°C

24.3 AIRWAY

Ensure that the airway is clear: the correct position for an infant for *all* resuscitation procedures is the neutral position. Both hyperextension and hypoextension of the neck will obstruct the airways. A prominent occiput will tend to flex the neck if the baby is placed dorsal on a flat surface, so it may be necessary to place a support below the baby's shoulders.

Deep suction of the airways should be avoided for at least 5 minutes after birth, except where there has been a history of meconium-stained amniotic fluid.

24.4 EVALUATION

The following three criteria should be evaluated in order (Figure 24.1):

- Breathing
- Heart rate
- Colour

24.5 BREATHING

If the airway is clear and effective breathing has not been established, then it will be necessary to provide oxygenation by means of assisted breaths. Weak respiratory efforts should be considered the same as no respiratory effort. Provide *five* inflation breaths to clear lung fluid. These are assisted breaths of about 30 cmH$_2$O for about 2–3 seconds. Once inflation breaths have been given, reassess the heart rate and colour. If the heart rate is increasing and the infant is pink, you have successfully inflated the lungs.

Reassess if effective breathing has not been established and/or the infant is not pink:

- Is the infant's airway clear?
- Are there chest movement when you provide ventilatory breaths?
- Has the heart rate picked up?

If the heart rate does not increase and the chest does not passively move with each inflation breath, then the airway is probably not clear, so confirm that the baby is in the neutral position and exclude an obstruction in the oropharynx.

If the heart rate remains slow (<60 bpm) or absent following five inflation breaths, despite good passive chest movement, start chest compression.

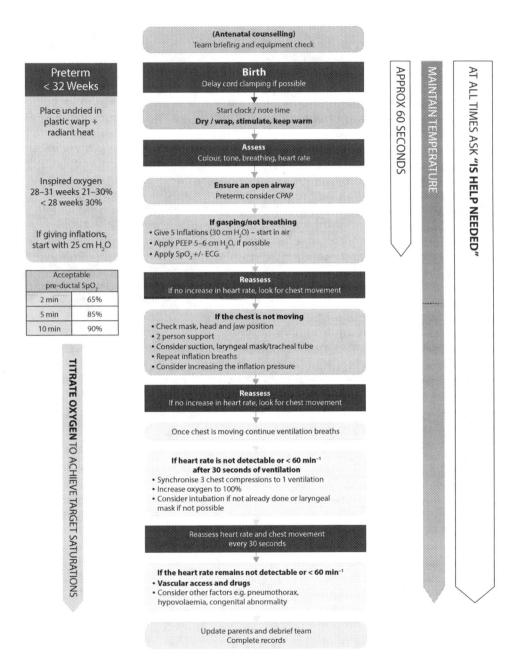

FIGURE 24.1   Newborn Life Support Algorithm 2021. Reproduced with permission from Resuscitation Council (UK). *Newborn resuscitation and support of transition of infants at birth 2021.* London: Resuscitation Council (UK), 2021.

24.6 CHEST COMPRESSION

In this event, chest compression will be necessary to support circulation until effective oxygenation and pulmonary blood flow are established.

- **Call for help** (paediatric assistance bleep . . .).
- Grip the chest in both hands, placing the thumbs together at the front and the fingers over the spine.
- Position the thumbs in the midline just below an imaginary line joining the nipples.
- Compress the chest, aiming to halve the distance between the sternum and the spine.
- Pause briefly between each compression. Aim for 40–60 compressions/min.
- Reassess heart rate every 30 seconds. Continue compression until the pulse rate is 80 beats/min.
- The conventional ratio is three compressions to one inflation breath.
- Increase oxygen to 100%.
- If there is no response to adequate compression and lung inflation, then it may be necessary to administer drugs via an umbilical venous catheter (standard doses of adrenaline given via the tracheal tube are unlikely to be as effective). Intraosseous route is also effective. If vascular access is not available and the baby is intubated, intrathecal route should be used.

Usually, drugs are required only in the most critically distressed infant. See the next section.

- Midwives may administer only vitamin K and naloxone (patient group directions).
- Check umbilical cord blood gases.
- Consider other factors, e.g. pneumothorax, hypovolaemia, congenital abnormality.

24.7 DRUGS USED IN NEONATAL RESUSCITATION

24.7.1 Adrenaline (1:10,000 solution)

- Dose: IV 20 micrograms per kg (0.2 mL/kg of 1:10,000 adrenaline [1000 micrograms in 10 mL]).
- Intra-tracheal route: 100 micrograms per kg (1.0 mL kg^{-1} of 1:10,000 adrenaline).
- If heart rate remains <60/min, additional doses may be given every 3–5 minutes.
- *Note*: 1:10,000 adrenaline = 1000 micrograms in 10 mL.

24.7.2 Glucose (10%)

Dose: IV 250 mg/kg bolus (2.5 mL/kg of 10% glucose).

24.7.3 Sodium bicarbonate (ideally 4.2% solution)

Dose: 1–2 mmol/kg (2–4 mL/kg of 4.2% solution) by slow intravenous injection.

24.8 VOLUME REPLACEMENT

If there is evidence that the baby has lost blood (or has shock unresponsive to other resuscitative measures), isotonic crystalloid may be needed, to increase cardiac output.

IV or intraosseous: 10 mL/kg of group O Rh-negative blood or isotonic crystalloid.

COMMUNICATION:

Keep the parent(s) posted on developments and interventions

Babies born before arrival at hospital

25

Babies born before arrival at hospital have relatively high morbidity rates owing to immaturity and low birth weight. *The main risk, irrespective of birth weight, is hypothermia.*

Some deliveries without medical or midwifery assistance take place at home. These should be managed according to local protocol, and transfer to hospital is not always necessary. Others will happen on the way to hospital or elsewhere outside the home.

There may be *background psychosocial problems*, which should be addressed where possible. In some cases, the pregnancy has been concealed or there has been no antenatal care.

25.1 MOTHER

- Check: Has the placenta been delivered? Is it complete?
- Assess the uterus for retraction
- Check for PPH
- Check for genital tract lacerations needing repair
- Check BP, pulse and temperature
- Check for any other obstetric, medical or social problems

25.2 BABY

- **Ensure that the baby is warm**
- Check colour, breathing and heart rate; call the paediatrician if indicated
- Check the gestational age
- Weigh the baby
- Administer vitamin K, with the mother's consent

Subsequent care as indicated.

DOI: 10.1201/9781315099897-28

Episiotomy

26

Indications for episiotomy include:

- Preventive action when a perineal tear is imminent
- Expedition of delivery in cases of fetal distress or maternal exhaustion
- Instrumental delivery
- Shoulder dystocia

Episiotomy should not be offered *routinely* at vaginal birth following previous third- or fourth-degree trauma.

Both the indication for episiotomy and the woman's assent should be documented in the labour records. A right mediolateral incision should be used (a midline incision increases the danger of damage to the anal sphincter).

Midwives who have been instructed in perineal repair may undertake the suturing of first- and second-degree tears and episiotomies using 2/0 Vicryl Rapide as suture material. The perineum is infiltrated with 1% lidocaine, the total amount not exceeding 20 mL.

Episiotomies should be repaired as soon as possible after completion of the third stage of labour, preferably by the person who has delivered the baby. Subcuticular suturing is preferable to interrupted suturing of the perineal skin, since it is associated with less pain.

For guidelines on the repair of perineal tears, see Chapter 48.

The following should be documented:

- The extent of the tear
- The type of suture
- Vaginal and rectal examination at the end of the procedure
- The swabs, sharps and instruments counted at the end of the procedure, and the fact that they are complete

---

EVOLVING PRACTICE

In the USA (where a midline episiotomy is cut), the rate of episiotomy with all vaginal deliveries decreased from 60.9% in 1979 to 24.5% in 2004 and 8% in 2017. Anal sphincter laceration with spontaneous vaginal delivery declined from 5% in 1979 to 3.5% in 2004.

DOI: 10.1201/9781315099897-29

The woman with a history of childhood sexual abuse

27

27.1 GENERAL MEASURES

- Give reassurance
- Provide the woman with a sense of control
- Assure her that you will respect her wishes
- The presence of a support person can be very helpful

27.2 COMMUNICATION

Choose your words carefully. Some words may bring back sad memories. Maintain confidentiality.

27.3 PHYSICAL EXAMINATION AND PROCEDURES

- Minimize internal examinations
- Find out if anything can be done to make the examination or procedure less stressful. For example, the woman may wish to take up a particular position or avoid the dorsal position
- Maintain utmost privacy during internal examinations
- Let the woman know that she can stop the examination or procedure at any time if she finds it too uncomfortable
- Handle the following with extra sensitivity:
  - Performing an episiotomy
  - Repairing an episiotomy or tear
  - Lithotomy position

DOI: 10.1201/9781315099897-30

27.4 FLASHBACKS

These may manifest as a panic attack, hyperventilation, a facial expression or a subtle change in body language. Be alert to nonverbal cues.

Use of birthing pool

28

The birthing pool may be used for one or both of the following:

- Immersion during the active phase of labour
- Delivery of the baby under water

Some women may feel a therapeutic benefit from immersion during labour, but delivery under water carries uncommon but significant risks to the baby, including drowning, respiratory problems, bleeding from a ruptured cord and waterborne infection.

Women using the birthing pool should be looked after only by midwives who have acquired the requisite skills and confidence.

28.1 INCLUSION CRITERIA

- 37 completed weeks
- Normal pregnancy
- Singleton fetus with cephalic presentation
- No systemic sedation
- Spontaneous rupture of membranes <24 hours
- Normal observations: pulse, temperature and BP
- Normal CTG

28.2 EXCLUSION CRITERIA

- APH
- Induction of labour
- Meconium-stained amniotic fluid
- IUGR
- Multiple pregnancy
- Malpresentation
- Previous CS
- Medical conditions: diabetes, epilepsy, HIV, group B streptococcus, etc.
- Any condition requiring continuous fetal monitoring
- Mother requiring IV cannula
- Macrosomic baby

DOI: 10.1201/9781315099897-31

- Opioid analgesia taken in the last 2 hours
- Suspected or confirmed COVID-19

28.3 CONDUCT OF LABOUR

28.3.1 The pool

- The water depth should be such that the woman's torso is exposed (i.e. not immersed), to facilitate thermoregulation through evaporation.
- The water should be free of debris during delivery.
- The floor of the pool room should be dry.
- The temperature should not exceed 37.5°C. Check the temperature of the pool hourly in the first stage of labour and quarter-hourly during second stage. Aim for a pool temperature of 32–36°C during labour and 36–37°C at delivery.
- Check the temperature of the woman hourly. If her temperature increases by 1°C above the baseline recording, she should be advised to leave the pool. Fetal temperature is slightly higher than the maternal temperature and raised maternal temperature could induce fetal tachycardia.

28.3.2 Analgesia

Entonox may be used. If pethidine or an epidural is required, the mother will have to leave the pool.

28.3.3 Progress of labour

- Monitor the fetal heart rate using underwater Doppler ultrasound.
- Vaginal examinations should be performed out of the pool.
- Progress should be recorded on the partogram.

28.4 SUPPORT IN LABOUR

- The woman should not be left on her own at any time.
- Give liberal oral fluids and avoid dehydration.

28.5 INDICATIONS FOR ASKING THE WOMAN TO LEAVE THE POOL

- Water temperature too hot or cold
- Elevated maternal temperature or abnormal vital signs
- Fetal heart rate abnormality

- Slow progress in first or second stage of labour
- Excessive bleeding
- Opioid or regional analgesia required
- Short umbilical cord

28.6 DELIVERY

- Two midwives should be present at delivery.
- If the woman raises herself out of the water and exposes the fetal head to air, once the presenting part is visible, she should be advised to remain out of the water to avoid the risk of premature gasping under water.
- Do not perform an episiotomy or cut the cord under water.
- If the baby is delivered in water, ensure that the head is the first part to emerge from the water and ensure that it does not go back under the water.

The cord should never be clamped or cut while the head is still under water.

- The third stage, whether active or physiological, must be performed out of water.

28.7 GENERAL

The usual infection control, handling and moving, and health and safety standards apply. Local protocols should be agreed with the microbiology and relevant governance teams. This includes guidance on the prevention of *Legionella* build-up in the water supply, particularly in seldomly used pools.

Further reading for Part II

Intravenous Cannulation

Niesen KM, Harris DY, Parkin LS, Henn LT. The effects of heparin versus normal saline for maintenance of peripheral intravenous locks in pregnant women. *J Obstet Gynecol Neonatal Nurs*. 2003;32(4):503–8. doi: 10.1177/0884217503255203

Prelabour rupture of membranes at term (37–42 weeks)

Mbaluka CM, Kamau K, Karanja JG, Mugo N. Effectiveness and safety of 2-hourly 20mcg oral misoprostol solution compared to standard intravenous oxytocin in labour induction due to pre-labour rupture of the membranes at term: A randomized clinical trial at Kenyatta national hospital. *East Afr Med J*. 2014;91(9):303–10

Middleton P, Shepherd E, Flenady V, McBain RD, Crowther CA. Planned early birth versus expectant management (waiting) for prelabour rupture of membranes at term (37 weeks or more). *Cochrane Database Syst Rev*. 2017;1(1):CD005302. doi: 10.1002/14651858.CD005302.pub3

Padayachee L, Kale M, Mannerfeldt J, Metcalfe A. Oral misoprostol for induction of labour in term PROM: A systematic review. *J Obstet Gynaecol Can*. 2020;42(12):1525–31.e1. doi: 10.1016/j.jogc.2020.02.111

Wojcieszek AM, Stock OM, Flenady V. Antibiotics for prelabour rupture of membranes at or near term. *Cochrane Database Syst Rev*. 2014;(10):CD001807. doi: 10.1002/14651858.CD001807.pub2

Management of the first stage of labour

Bohren MA, Hofmeyr GJ, Sakala C, Fukuzawa RK, Cuthbert A. Continuous support for women during childbirth. *Cochrane Database Syst Rev*. 2017;7(7):CD003766. doi: 10.1002/14651858.CD003766.pub6

Caldeyro-Barcia R, Noriega-Guerra L, Cibils LA, et al. Effect of position changes on the intensity and frequency of uterine contractions during labor. *Am J Obstet Gynecol*. 1960; 80:284–90

Lawrence A, Lewis L, Hofmeyr GJ, Styles C. Maternal positions and mobility during first stage labour. *Cochrane Database Syst Rev*. 2013;10:CD003934. doi: 10.1002/14651858.CD003934.pub4

National Institute for Health and Clinical Excellence (NICE). *Intrapartum Care for Healthy Women and Babies*. Clinical Guideline [CG190] Published 2014 Dec, Last updated 2017 Feb

Providing Oral Nutrition to Women in Labor. American college of nurse-midwives. *J Midwifery Womens Health*. 2016;61(4):528–34. doi: 10.1111/jmwh.12515

Fetal monitoring

Alfirevic Z, Devane D, Gyte GM, Cuthbert A. Continuous cardiotocography (CTG) as a form of electronic fetal monitoring (EFM) for fetal assessment during labour. *Cochrane Database Syst Rev*. 2017;2(2):CD006066. doi: 10.1002/14651858.CD006066.pub3

Gibb D, Arulkumaran S. *Fetal Monitoring in Practice*, 4th edn. Edinburgh: Churchill Livingstone, 2017

Knupp RJ, Andrews WW, Tita ATN. The future of electronic fetal monitoring. *Best Pract Res Clin Obstet Gynaecol*. 2020;67:44–52. doi: 10.1016/j.bpobgyn.2020.02.004

Martis R, Emilia O, Nurdiati DS, Brown J. Intermittent auscultation (IA) of fetal heart rate in labour for fetal well-being. *Cochrane Database Syst Rev*. 2017;2(2):CD008680. doi: 10.1002/14651858.CD008680.pub2

National Institute for Health and Care Excellence. *Intrapartum Care*. NICE Guideline CG190 NICE, February 2017

DOI: 10.1201/9781315099897-32

Fetal scalp blood sampling

Gilbert M, Ghesquiere L, Drumez E, Subtil D, Fague V, Berveiller P, Garabedian C. How to reduce fetal scalp blood sampling? A retrospective study evaluating the diagnostic value of scalp stimulation to predict fetal wellbeing assessed by scalp blood sampling. *Eur J Obstet Gynecol Reprod Biol.* 2021;263:153–8. doi: 10.1016/j.ejogrb.2021.05.032

Jørgensen JS, Weber T. Fetal scalp blood sampling in labor – a review. *Acta Obstet Gynecol Scand.* 2014;93(6):548–55. doi: 10.1111/aogs.12421

Pascual Mancho J, Marti Gamboa S, Redrado Gimenez O, Crespo Esteras R, Rodriguez Solanilla B, Castan Mateo S. Diagnostic accuracy of fetal scalp lactate for intrapartum acidosis compared with scalp pH. *J Perinat Med.* 2017;45(3):315–20. doi: 10.1515/jpm-2016-0044

Prouhèze A, Girault A, Barrois M, Lepercq J, Goffinet F, Le Ray C. Fetal scalp blood sampling: Do pH and lactates provide the same information? *J Gynecol Obstet Hum Reprod.* 2021;50(4):101964. doi: 10.1016/j.jogoh.2020.101964

Augmentation of labour

Cheek TG, Samuels P, Miller F, et al. Normal saline i.v. fluid decreases uterine activity in active labour. *Br J Anaesth.* 1996;77:632–5

Dawood F, Dowswell T, Quenby S. Intravenous fluids for reducing the duration of labour in low risk nulliparous women. *Cochrane Database Syst Rev.* 2013;(6):CD007715. doi: 10.1002/14651858.CD007715.pub2

Patka JH, Lodolce AE, Johnston AK. High-versus low-dose oxytocin for augmentation or induction of labor. *Ann Pharmacother.* 2005;39:95–101

Smyth RMD, Markham C, Dowswell T. Amniotomy for shortening spontaneous labour. *Cochrane Database Syst Rev.* 2013;6. Art. No:CD006167. doi: 10.1002/14651858.CD006167.pub4

Epidural analgesia in labour

Association of Anaesthetists of Great Britain & Ireland, Obstetric Anaesthetists' Association. *OAA/AAGBI Guidelines for Obstetric Anaesthetic Services 2013.* London: AAGBI and OAA, June 2013. Available at: www.obstetric_anaesthetic_services_2013.pdf (oaa-anaes.ac.uk)

Horlocker TT, Heit JA. Low molecular weight heparin: Biochemistry, pharmacology, peri-operative prophylaxis regimens, and guidelines for regional anaesthetic management. *Anesth Analg.* 1997;85:874–85

Ronel I, Weiniger CF. Non-regional analgesia for labour: Remifentanil in obstetrics. *BJA Educ.* 2019;19(11):357–61. doi:10.1016/j.bjae.2019.07.002

Roofthooft E, Barbé A, Schildermans J, Cromheecke S, Devroe S, Fieuws S, Rex S, Wong CA, Van de Velde M. Programmed intermittent epidural bolus vs. patient-controlled epidural analgesia for maintenance of labour analgesia: A two-centre, double-blind, randomised study†. *Anaesthesia.* 2020;75(12):1635–42. doi: 10.1111/anae.15149. Erratum in: *Anaesthesia.* 2021 Apr;76(4):567

Russell R. Preeclampsia and the anaesthesiologist: Current management. *Curr Opin Anaesthesiol.* 2020 Jun;33(3):305–10. doi: 10.1097/ACO.0000000000000835

Sng BL, Sia ATH. Maintenance of epidural labour analgesia: The old, the new and the future. *Best Pract Res Clin Anaesthesiol.* 2017;31(1):15–22. doi: 10.1016/j.bpa.2017.01.002

Management of the second stage of labour

Altman M, Lydon-Rochelle M. Prolonged second stage of labor and the risk of adverse maternal and perinatal outcomes: A systematic review. *Birth.* 2006;33:315–22

Di Mascio D, Saccone G, Bellussi F, Al-Kouatly HB, Brunelli R, Benedetti Panici P, Liberati M, D'Antonio F, Berghella V. Delayed versus immediate pushing in the second stage of labor in women with neuraxial analgesia: A systematic review and meta-analysis of randomized controlled trials. *Am J Obstet Gynecol.* 2020;223(2):189–203. doi: 10.1016/j.ajog.2020.02.002

Gimovsky AC, Berghella V. Prolonged second stage: What is the optimal length? *Obstet Gynecol Surv.* 2016;71(11):667–74. doi: 10.1097/OGX.0000000000000368

Lemos A, Amorim MM, Dornelas de Andrade A, de Souza AI, Cabral Filho JE, Correia JB. Pushing/bearing down methods for the second stage of labour. *Cochrane Database Syst Rev.* 2017;3(3):CD009124. doi: 10.1002/14651858.CD009124.pub3

Management of the third stage of labour

Begley CM, Gyte GM, Devane D, McGuire W, Weeks A, Biesty LM. Active versus expectant management for women in the third stage of labour. *Cochrane Database Syst Rev*. 2019;2(2):CD007412. doi: 10.1002/14651858. CD007412.pub5

Clebak KT, Croad JR, Lutzkanin AI. Active vs. expectant management in the third stage of labor. *Am Fam Physician*. 2021 Apr 1;103(7):404–5

Oladapo OT, Okusanya BO, Abalos E, Gallos ID, Papadopoulou A. Intravenous versus intramuscular prophylactic oxytocin for the third stage of labour. *Cochrane Database Syst Rev*. 2020;11(11):CD009332. doi: 10.1002/14651858.CD009332.pub4

Weeks AD, Fawcus S. Management of the third stage of labour: (For the optimal intrapartum care series edited by Mercedes Bonet, Femi Oladapo and Metin Gülmezoglu). *Best Pract Res Clin Obstet Gynaecol*. 2020;67:65–79. doi: 10.1016/j.bpobgyn.2020.03.003

Immediate postpartum care

Christensson K, Siles C, Moreno L, et al. Temperature, metabolic adaptation and crying in healthy full-term newborns cared for skin-to-skin or in a cot. *Acta Paediatr*. 1992;81:488–93

Moore ER, Bergman N, Anderson GC, Medley N. Early skin-to-skin contact for mothers and their healthy newborn infants. *Cochrane Database Syst Rev*. 2016;11(11):CD003519. doi: 10.1002/14651858.CD003519.pub4

Care of the newborn

Fawke J, et al. Newborn resuscitation and support of transition of infants at birth guidelines. *Resuscitation*. 2021 May;161:291

Jullien S. Vitamin K prophylaxis in newborns. *BMC Pediatr*. 2021;21(Suppl 1):350. doi: 10.1186/s12887-021-02701-4

Sankar MJ, Chandrasekaran A, Kumar P, Thukral A, Agarwal R, Paul VK. Vitamin K prophylaxis for prevention of vitamin K deficiency bleeding: A systematic review. *J Perinatol*. 2016;36(Suppl 1):S29–35. doi: 10.1038/jp.2016.30

Meconium-stained amniotic fluid

Foster JP, Dawson JA, Davis PG, Dahlen HG. Routine oro/nasopharyngeal suction versus no suction at birth. *Cochrane Database Syst Rev*. 2017;4(4):CD010332. doi: 10.1002/14651858.CD010332.pub2

Kelly LE, Shivananda S, Murthy P, Srinivasjois R, Shah PS. Antibiotics for neonates born through meconium-stained amniotic fluid. *Cochrane Database Syst Rev*. 2017;6(6):CD006183. doi: 10.1002/14651858. CD006183.pub2

Nangia S, Thukral A, Chawla D. Tracheal suction at birth in non-vigorous neonates born through meconium-stained amniotic fluid. *Cochrane Database Syst Rev*. 2021 Jun 16;6(6):CD012671. doi: 10.1002/14651858.CD012671. pub2

Phattraprayoon N, Tangamornsuksan W, Ungtrakul T. Outcomes of endotracheal suctioning in non-vigorous neonates born through meconium-stained amniotic fluid: A systematic review and meta-analysis. *Arch Dis Child Fetal Neonatal Ed*. 2021 Jan;106(1):31–8. doi: 10.1136/archdischild-2020-318941

Vain NE, Szyld EG, Prudent LM, et al. Oropharyngeal and nasopharyngeal suctioning of meconium-stained neonates before delivery of their shoulders: Multicentre, randomised controlled trial. *Lancet*. 2004;364:597–602

Wiswell TE, Gannon CM, Jacob J, et al. Delivery room management of the apparently vigorous meconium-stained neonate: Results of the multicenter international collaborative trial. *Pediatric*. 2000;105:1–7

Xu H, Mas-Calvet M, Wei SQ, Luo ZC, Fraser WD. Abnormal fetal heart rate tracing patterns in patients with thick meconium staining of the amniotic fluid: Association with perinatal outcomes. *Am J Obstet Gynecol*. 2009;200:283.e1–7

Neonatal resuscitation

Berkelhamer SK, Kamath-Rayne BD, Niermeyer S. Neonatal resuscitation in low-resource settings. *Clin Perinatol*. 2016;43(3):573–91. doi: 10.1016/j.clp.2016.04.013

Hainstock LM, Raval GR. Neonatal resuscitation. *Pediatr Rev*. 2020;41(3):155–8. doi: 10.1542/pir.2018-0203

Richmond S. Newborn life support. In: *Resuscitation Guidelines 2005*. Resuscitation Council UK, December 2005:97–104. Available at: www.resus.org.uk/pages/nls.pdf

Trevisanuto D, Galderisi A. Neonatal resuscitation: State of the art. *Am J Perinatol*. 2019;36(Suppl 2):S29–32. doi: 10.1055/s-0039-1691797

Babies born before arrival at hospital

Bhoopalam PS, Watkinson M. Babies born before arrival at hospital. *Br J Obstet Gynaecol*. 1991;98:57–64

Boland RA, Davis PG, Dawson JA, Stewart MJ, Smith J, Doyle LW. Very preterm birth before arrival at hospital. *Aust N Z J Obstet Gynaecol*. 2018;58(2):197–203. doi: 10.1111/ajo.1269

Hadar A, Rabinovich A, Sheiner E, Landau D, Hallak M, Mazor M. Obstetric characteristics and neonatal outcome of unplanned out-of-hospital term deliveries: A prospective, case-control study. *J Reprod Med*. 2005;50(11):832–6

Rodie VA, Thomson AJ, Norman JE. Accidental out-of-hospital deliveries: An obstetric and neonatal case control study. *Acta Obstet Gynecol Scand*. 2002;81:50–4

Repair of episiotomy and first-/second-degree perineal repair

Kettle C, Dowswell T, Ismail KM. Continuous and interrupted suturing techniques for repair of episiotomy or second-degree tears. *Cochrane Database Syst Rev*. 2012;11(11):CD000947. doi: 10.1002/14651858.CD000947.pub3

The woman with a history of childhood sexual abuse

Leeners B, Neumaier-Wagner P, Quarg AF, Rath W. Childhood sexual abuse (CSA) experiences: An underestimated factor in perinatal care. *Acta Obstet Gynecol Scand*. 2006;85:971–6

Leeners B, Richter-Appelt H, Imthurn B, Rath W. Influence of childhood sexual abuse on pregnancy, delivery, and the early postpartum period in adult women. *J Psychosom Res*. 2006;61:139–51

Rhodes N, Hutchinson S. Labor experiences of childhood sexual abuse survivors. *Birth*. 1994;21:213–20

Sobel L, O'Rourke-Suchoff D, Holland E, Remis K, Resnick K, Perkins R, Bell S. Pregnancy and childbirth after sexual trauma: Patient perspectives and care preferences. *Obstet Gynecol*. 2018;132(6):1461–8. doi: 10.1097/AOG.0000000000002956

Use of birthing pool

Bovbjerg ML, Cheyney M, Everson C. Maternal and newborn outcomes following waterbirth: The midwives alliance of North America statistics project, 2004 to 2009 cohort. *J Midwifery Womens Health*. 2016;61(1):11–20. doi: 10.1111/jmwh.12394

Cluett ER, Burns E, Cuthbert A. Immersion in water during labour and birth (Cochrane Review). *Cochrane Database Syst Rev*. 2018;5(5):CD000111. doi: 10.1002/14651858.CD000111

Royal College of Obstetricians and Gynaecologists/Royal College of Midwives Joint statement No.1: Immersion in water during labour and birth. London; RCOG 2006. http://activebirthpools.com/wp-content/uploads/2014/05/RCOG-waterbirth.pdf

PART III

Abnormal and high-risk labour

Formal risk assessment and contingency planning should start antenatally – but should not end there. Each clinical episode offers an opportunity to reassess and contain risk.

DOI: 10.1201/9781315099897-33

SECTION 1

Powers, passenger, passage

Caesarean section

29

29.1 PREPARATIONS

- Obtain consent. A competent pregnant woman is entitled to decline CS, even if her life or that of the baby is at risk.
- Group-and-save or cross-match, as required. Blood should be cross-matched if any of the following apply:
  - Maternal anaemia ([Hb] <10 g/dL)
  - Placenta praevia (cross-match 4 units)
  - Anterior placenta and previous CS
  - Any other situation where higher than usual blood loss is anticipated (e.g. a clotting disorder or large fibroids)
- Insert a cannula (size 16G).
- Perform a risk assessment for DVT prophylaxis.
- Ensure the woman has fasted for at least 6 hours before an elective CS. She may drink water (150 mL) up to 2 hours before elective surgery.
- In the case of CS for breech presentation (elective or emergency), confirm by means of an ultrasound scan that the presentation is still breech.

In theatre:

- Catheterize the bladder (if not already done).
- Check fetal heart tones.
- Place the patient in the left lateral tilt (15°).

29.2 MEDICATION TO REDUCE THE RISK OF ASPIRATION SYNDROME

- Ranitidine 150 mg orally on the night of admission and at 0730 the following day. For emergencies, check whether ranitidine was given in labour (oral ranitidine 150 mg is effective if given at least 60 minutes before CS). If not, give ranitidine 50 mg in 20 mL 0.9% saline IV, over 2 minutes.
- Metoclopramide 10 mg orally.
- Sodium citrate 30 mL orally.

29.3 CLASSIFICATION OF URGENCY OF CS

- **Emergency – to be performed immediately**:
  - Immediate threat to life of woman or fetus
  - Massive APH
  - Cord prolapse
  - Placental abruption
  - Profound unresponsive fetal bradycardia
  - Fetal distress (pH ≤ 7.20)
  - Uterine rupture
- **Urgent**: maternal or fetal compromise that is not immediately life-threatening (e.g. failure to progress).
- **Scheduled**: needing early delivery but no immediate maternal or fetal compromise (e.g. IUGR with abnormal Doppler).
- **Elective**: at a time to suit the woman and the maternity team, e.g. previous CS.

When CS becomes a probability for a woman in labour, she should be informed and the anaesthetist should be alerted. This may allow discussion with the woman in less pressing circumstances.

29.4 ELECTIVE CS

- To reduce the risk of respiratory distress in the newborn, elective CS should not be performed routinely before 39 weeks' gestation. In selected cases, it will be sensible to schedule the operation earlier than this. For example, it may be safer to have a planned CS at 38 weeks for a woman with placenta praevia or three previous CS than have this woman present in labour a few days before a CS booked for 39 weeks.
- Book with the labour ward as directed by local protocol.
- There should be a maximum of three cases per 3.5-hour operating session (two cases, if complicated).
- If the woman falls into any of the following categories, the list should be covered by the consultant anaesthetist:
  - Previous anaesthetic complications
  - Obesity (body mass index >30 kg/m^2 at booking)
  - Multiple pregnancy
  - Placenta praevia
  - Hypertensive disease
  - Diabetes mellitus
  - Jehovah's Witness
  - Significant coexisting disease (cardiac, renal or respiratory)
- Low-risk patients can be admitted on the day of operation, but bloods and consent must be obtained in clinic, ranitidine prescribed, and the patient told to fast from midnight.

29.5 WORKPLACE NOISE

'Noise hygiene' should be maintained. Side conversations among staff should be avoided, especially if the woman is awake and/or her partner is present in the operating room.

Bleeps should not be brought into the operating theatre. If a bleep goes off in theatre during induction of general anaesthesia or while the patient is under regional analgesia, it could be alarming to the patient and/or her partner. There could also be breach of confidentiality when messages are passed to the doctor.

29.6 EMERGENCY CS

- Contact the consultant on duty/call (in their absence, contact any other consultant)
- Obtain consent
- Classify and document the urgency of the operation (see the aforementioned classification)
- Notify:
  - The operating department practitioner (ODP)
  - The anaesthetist (specify the urgency of the operation)
  - The paediatrician
- FBC, group-and-save or cross-match as required
- Discontinue Syntocinon (oxytocin) infusion, if in progress
- Ensure that thromboprophylaxis is administered

29.7 SURGICAL PROCEDURE

- The procedure is performed with the patient in a left lateral tilt.
  - The woman should be accorded due respect and dignity throughout the operation. This means, for example, that she is unclothed only as and when necessary, noise and frivolous side conversations are minimized, and the operation field is screened from view. Her partner should also be supported.
  - Do not exteriorize the uterus as routine.
  - Allow spontaneous separation of the placenta followed by cord traction. This is preferable to manual removal of the placenta. Manual removal is associated with increased blood loss and postpartum endometritis.
- Cord blood gas analysis should be performed following CS for fetal distress.
- Administer prophylactic antibiotics.

29.8 PROPHYLACTIC ANTIBIOTICS

Antibiotics given prophylactically reduce the incidence of postpartum endometritis.

The antibiotic is administered after the umbilical cord has been clamped: cefuroxime IV 750 mg and metronidazole IV 500 mg immediately.

If the woman is allergic to penicillin, then give erythromycin 1 g.

For prophylactic antibiotic regime in specific situations, e.g. cardiac disease, see the relevant chapter in this book.

29.9 HIGH-RISK CASES

A consultant or suitably experienced senior doctor should be present for CS performed for the following indications/circumstances:

- Placenta praevia
- Placental abruption
- Multiple previous CS
- Body mass index >35 kg/m^2
- Delivery <32 weeks
- Any other potentially complicated CS

29.10 DELAYED ELECTIVE CS

- Keep the woman and her partner informed of events.
- If the operation is delayed by more than 4 hours, start an IV infusion.

29.11 POSTOPERATIVE CARE

The woman should be monitored by an appropriately trained member of staff until she is stable and able to communicate. See Chapter 30.

Respiratory rate, heart rate, BP, pain and sedation should be recorded every half-hour for 4 hours, then 4-hourly. The use of an EWS chart is recommended.

If CS was done under regional block, the indwelling bladder catheter should remain in place until the woman is ambulant, to prevent bladder over-distension.

Give analgesia as required.

29.12 THROMBOPROPHYLAXIS

Ensure that thromboprophylaxis has been prescribed/administered. LMWH can be commenced 6 hours after spinal anaesthesia, and 8 hours after epidural analgesia.

- Pressure stockings should be worn
- Ensure adequate hydration
- Mobilise early

Recovery of obstetric patients

30

All patients should be recovered in a designated fully staffed and equipped recovery area. They should be under continuous clinical observation for at least 30 minutes:

- Continuous ECG
- Pulse oximetry
- BP monitoring

The following should be documented:

- Level of consciousness
- Pulse rate
- Temperature
- Pain score
- BP
- O_2 saturation and O_2 administration
- Respiratory rate
- Blood loss from wound (and from drain, if present)
- IV infusions
- Blood loss from vagina
- Urine output and colour
- Drugs administered: analgesia
- VTE prophylaxis: Flotron; LMWH
- Check of epidural site

The frequency of observations will depend on the stage of recovery and the clinical condition of the patient, but vital signs should be recorded at least every 15 minutes in the first hour.

Discharge from the recovery area should be according to a protocol agreed by the anaesthetist.

Before transfer to the postnatal ward, all patients must:

- Be easily rousable
- Have full airway control
- Have adequate pain relief
- Have normal observations
- Have IV fluids, antiemetics and analgesia prescribed as required

Post-recovery care:

- Continue observation of vital signs as specified in local protocol.
- Encourage deep breathing, coughing and leg exercises.
- Assist with breastfeeding.
- Ambulate within 6–12 hours.

DOI: 10.1201/9781315099897-36

! Midwifery staff deputed to look after postoperative patients should be specifically trained in monitoring, care of the airway and resuscitative procedures and should be supervised by a defined anaesthetist at all times.

UK Health Departments. *Report on Confidential Enquiries into Maternal Deaths in the United Kingdom 1988–1990.* London: HMSO, 1994

High-dependency care

31

High-dependency care is indicated in the following circumstances:

- When there is haemodynamic instability (due to hypovolaemia, haemorrhage or sepsis)
- When a continuous ECG is required
- For invasive pressure monitoring (central venous pressure or arterial line)
- When there is acute impairment of respiratory, renal or metabolic function

One or more of the above is likely to happen in cases of:

- Major PPH
- Fulminating pre-eclampsia
- Eclampsia
- DIC
- Pulmonary oedema
- Cardiac failure
- Cardiomyopathy
- Sudden maternal collapse
- Septicaemia

All observations and results of investigations must be recorded in a high-dependency chart.

Some patients may need to be transferred to the general HDU or ICU of the hospital. This should be done in consultation with both the consultant anaesthetist and the consultant obstetrician. Timely transfer to ICU is associated with a better outcome; conversely, delayed transfer has contributed to maternal death in some cases reviewed by the *Confidential Enquiries into Maternal Deaths in the United Kingdom*.

31.1 EARLY WARNING SCORE

Observational studies show that obstetric early warning charts are useful in predicting obstetric morbidity and mortality.

An example of an EWS grid is provided in Table 31.1. The selection of cases, frequency of recording and whom to call for various levels of EWS should be according to local protocols.

DOI: 10.1201/9781315099897-37

TABLE 31.1   A Matrix for Determining Early Warning Score

SCORE	3	2	1	0	1	2	3
Temp	–	≤35.0	35.1–36.0	36.1–37.9	38.0–38.9	≥39.0	–
Systolic BP	≤70	71–80	81–100	101–139	–	140–159	≥160
Diastolic BP	–	–	–	<90	90–109	–	≥110
HR	–	≤40	41–50	51–100	101–110	111–129	≥130
RR	–	≤8	–	9–14	15–20	21–29	≥30
CNS	–	–	–	Alert	Voice	Pain	Unresponsive
%SaO$_2$	–	–	–	–	–	–	≤92 air or ≤95 in O$_2$

EWS = 6: High risk of deterioration
EWS = 4–5: Medium risk of deterioration
EWS = 3: Low risk of deterioration

Note: Scores between 3 and 6 should trigger action as directed in the local protocol. For a statistically based, internally validated obstetric EWS, see: Carle C, Alexander P, Columb M, Johal J. Design and internal validation of an obstetric early warning score: Secondary analysis of the Intensive Care National Audit and Research Centre Case Mix Programme database. Anaesthesia. 2013;68(4):354–67. doi:10.1111/anae.12180

Alert!

Early warning charts should be used *in conjunction with* clinical judgement.

Failed intubation drill

32

The incidence of failed intubation is higher in obstetric anaesthesia than in the general population. In one UK region, the incidence was 1 in 238 anaesthetics, and in half of the cases reviewed there was a failure to follow an accepted protocol for failed tracheal intubation.

There should be no more than two attempts at intubation. Repeated attempts increase the chances of aspiration. For the second attempt, use a bougie or smaller tracheal tubes and/or McCoy laryngoscope as appropriate. Failed intubation causes no harm to the mother if oxygenation is maintained.

- Call for help
- Maintain cricoid pressure
- Keep the patient in a supine position with left lateral tilt
- Give oxygen via a facemask
- If successful, await return of spontaneous ventilation, turn the woman and allow her to waken
- If mask ventilation is not possible, attempt insertion of a laryngeal mask airway (a supraglottic airway device). This will require partial release of cricoid pressure. No more than two attempts

If successful, turn the patient and either allow her to waken or proceed with surgery if imperative. Surgery should proceed only if the mother's life depends on it (e.g. in cardiac arrest or massive haemorrhage).

- If laryngeal mask airway insertion is unsuccessful and spontaneous breathing does not return, declare 'CICO' – can't intubate, can't oxygenate.
- Management of CICO:
  - Call ENT surgeon
  - Exclude laryngospasm. Ensure muscle paralysis before proceeding to FONA (front of neck airway)
  - Perform needle cricothyrotomy – Access the trachea through the cricothyroid membrane, which is located just superior to the 'Adam's apple'. There are other techniques of FONA

If FONA is successful, determine whether to wake her or proceed with surgery.

- If FONA is unsuccessful, proceed to perimortem CS and advanced life support.
- If expertise for FONA is not immediately available, consider CS under local anaesthetic.

At a UK hospital, emergency caesarean section for fetal distress was successfully performed under local anaesthesia in a 25-year-old primigravida with BMI of 49 after failed intubation, unsuccessful failed intubation drill and multiple failed attempts at combined spinal epidural analgesia (see 'Further reading' on p. 287).

DOI: 10.1201/9781315099897-38

Instrumental delivery

33

Approximately 1 in 10 deliveries in the industrialized world is an instrumental vaginal delivery. Instrumental delivery carries significant risks of acute and long-term physical and psychological complications for mother and baby. Care should be taken in selecting cases.

33.1 NON-OPERATIVE INTERVENTIONS WHICH REDUCE INSTRUMENTAL DELIVERY RATES

- One-to-one support in labour
- Upright or lateral position
- Oxytocin for prolonged second stage
- Delayed pushing for women using epidural analgesia

33.2 AVOIDING HARM

Harm can be avoided if precautions are taken:

- Following the advice given earlier to reduce the rate of instrumental delivery
- Careful case selection – knowing when and when not to perform forceps or vacuum-assisted (ventouse) delivery
- Appropriate pre-application assessment (see later)
- Use of the right technique
- Appropriate management of malrotation
- Appropriate management of trial of instrumental delivery
- Mindfulness – beware of fixation with achieving vaginal delivery

33.3 INDICATIONS FOR INSTRUMENTAL DELIVERY

- Fetal distress
- Maternal distress or exhaustion
- Delayed second stage of labour (see Chapter 18)
- After-coming head at breech delivery

DOI: 10.1201/9781315099897-39

- Elective procedure where maternal down-bearing effort is inadvisable:
  - Dural tap at epidural
  - Maternal heart disease
  - Severe pre-eclampsia
  - Respiratory distress
  - Detached retina

33.4 CONDITIONS TO BE FULFILLED BEFORE INSTRUMENTAL DELIVERY

- There is full cervical dilatation.
- The bladder has been catheterized.
- Presentation is cephalic.
- The bony presenting part is at or below the level of the ischial spines.
- No more than one-fifth of the fetal head is palpable abdominally.
- The position of the presenting part is defined clearly.
- The fetal membranes have ruptured.
- There is adequate analgesia.
- There are good uterine contractions.
- The pelvis is judged to be clinically adequate (subpubic arch; interspinous distance; moulding/caput).

It follows from the aforementioned that cephalopelvic disproportion, unengaged fetal head and malpresentation (e.g. brow or breech presentation) are contraindications to instrumental delivery. For further contraindications specific to vacuum-assisted delivery, see later.

33.5 CLASSIFICATION OF INSTRUMENTAL VAGINAL DELIVERY

The classification of instrumental vaginal delivery according to the American College of Obstetricians and Gynecologists (ACOG) is shown in Table 33.1.

33.6 COMMUNICATION

The woman (and her partner if present) should be kept informed before and during the procedure:

- Warn that an episiotomy may be performed.
- For vacuum-assisted delivery, warn to expect a temporary swelling on the baby's head where the cup is applied.

All women having an instrumental delivery should have a left lateral tilt to prevent supine hypotension syndrome.

TABLE 33.1   ACOG Classification of Instrumental Vaginal Delivery

Type	Indices
Outlet	• Fetal scalp is visible without separating the labia
	• Fetal skull has reached the pelvic floor
	• Sagittal suture is in the anteroposterior diameter or right or left
	• occiput anterior or posterior position (rotation ≤ 45°)
	• Fetal head is at or on the perineum
Low	• Leading point of the skull (not caput) is at station plus ≥2 cm and not on the pelvic floor
	• Two subdivisions:
	a. rotation ≤45°
	b. rotation >45°
Mid	• Fetal head is one-fifth palpable per abdomen
	• Leading point of the skull is above station plus 2 cm but not above the ischial spines
	• Two subdivisions:
	a. rotation ≤45°
	b. rotation >45°
High	Not included in classification

Source: Reproduced with permission from *Operative Vaginal Delivery, Technical Bulletin 196.* Washington, DC: *American College of Obstetricians and Gynecologists*

33.7 CHOICE OF INSTRUMENT

The operator should use an instrument that they are comfortable with.

Forceps should be used where vacuum-assisted delivery is contraindicated (see later). Forceps are also preferable if there is poor or no maternal effort (poor uterine action or the woman is too tired to push).

Do not use the vacuum extractor if gestational age <32 weeks; use with caution if 32–36 + 0 weeks.

33.8 PRE-APPLICATION ASSESSMENT: ABDOMINAL AND VAGINAL EXAMINATION

- Palpation of the abdomen
- Empty the bladder
- Cervical dilatation
- Position
- Station – The *bony* presenting part should be at or below the level of the ischial spines
- Moulding (moulding) – Risk of intracranial injury increases in severe moulding
- Synclitic or asynclitic
- Flexion

ALERT!

Moulding, caput and station

When assessing station of the fetal head, be aware that the longitudinal axis of the fetal head is elongated by moulding and caput. These may create the false impression that the (bony) presenting part is lower than it is.

See Figures 33.1 and 33.2.

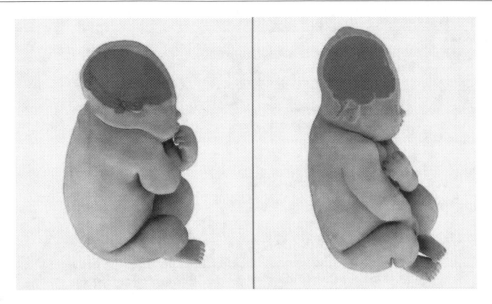

FIGURE 33.1   Elongation of the fetal head by moulding ± caput.

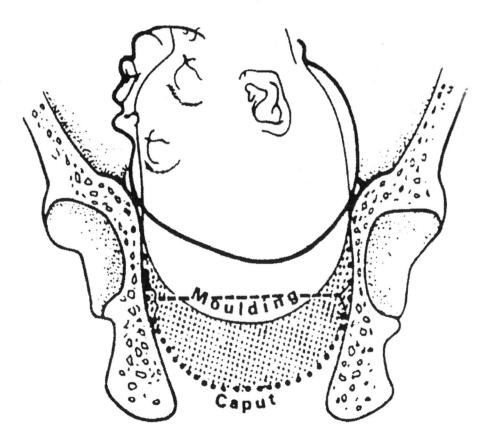

FIGURE 33.2   Caput and moulding may give the false impression that the bony presenting part is lower than it is (or that the widest presenting diameter has entered the pelvic brim.

Crichton D. A reliable method of establishing the level of the fetal head in obstetrics. S Afr Med J. 1974;12:784–7

33.9 VACUUM-ASSISTED DELIVERY

Choose the appropriate cup:

- Soft (silicone or plastic) cups should only be used for outlet deliveries and occipito-anterior position with ≤45° rotation.
- For other cases, use a rigid (plastic or metal) cup. For occipito-posterior and occipito-transverse positions, a rigid cup designed for posterior application should be used.

Whichever cup is used, the most important factor in accomplishing safe delivery is correct placement of the cup.

33.10 PROCEDURE

A: Ask for help, address the woman, palpate the abdomen and ensure that anaesthesia is adequate.
B: Bladder is empty.
C: Cervix is completely dilated.
D: Determine position.
E: Equipment is ready. Lubricate.
F: 'Flexing median' application of cup (Figure 33.3). The flexion point is located on the sagittal suture *3 cm in front of the posterior fontanelle*. Check the vacuum cup to ensure that it does not include maternal tissue.

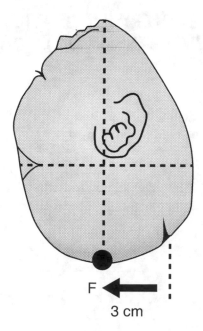

F ← 3 cm

FIGURE 33.3   The flexion point, located on the sagittal suture *3 cm in front of the posterior fontanelle*, is a key landmark in vacuum-assisted delivery because if the cup is not applied over this point, deflection of the head and cup detachment are more likely to occur. Sudden detachment may cause scalp injury. The sagittal suture should be centred under the vacuum.

G: Gentle, steady traction, should be applied at right angles to the cup, the axis of traction following the pelvic curve.

H: Halt the procedure if:
- There has been no descent with three consecutive pulls.
- The cup detaches two times, and the head is not on the perineum – cup detachment is associated with rapid compression/decompression forces and should be avoided.
- 15 minutes have elapsed since application of the cup (some protocols allow up to 20 minutes).

I: Evaluate for incision. Routine episiotomy is not necessary.

J: Remove the cup when the jaw is visible.

In the following cases, provided that there is no cephalopelvic disproportion, a senior, experienced obstetrician may opt to conduct a vacuum-assisted delivery when the cervix is 9 cm dilated, as the benefits outweigh the risk of injury to the cervix:

- Delivery of the second twin
- Cord prolapse
- Fetal distress with the presenting part below the level of the ischial spines

The case of *Fotedar v St George's Healthcare NHS Trust* [2005] EWHC 1327 (QB) concerned a child who sustained brain damage at birth following a vacuum-assisted delivery. The claimant maintained that a caesarean section should have been performed as the mother was not fully dilated and there was cephalo-pelvic disproportion. The High Court found the senior registrar negligent.

33.11 CONTRAINDICATIONS TO VACUUM-ASSISTED DELIVERY

- Fetal thrombocytopenia or clotting disorder
- Maternal idiopathic thrombocytopenic purpura
- Early preterm labour (<34 weeks) – vacuum should not be used, because of the risk of intracranial haemorrhage, cephalhaematoma and neonatal jaundice, but forceps may be applied
- Malpresentation (face or brow)
- Cephalopelvic disproportion
- Repeated scalp FBS
- Fetal head not engaged

33.12 FORCEPS DELIVERY

A–E: as above.

F: The forceps blades are applied and checked.
1. Check the posterior fontanelle – it should be one finger's breadth above the plane of the shanks (baby in OA position).

2. Check the sagittal suture – it should be perpendicular to the plane of the shanks.
3. Check the fenestration – the space at the heel of the forceps should admit a fingertip only.

G: Gentle traction should be applied, as described earlier. Ease the grip between contractions to reduce compression of the baby's head.

H: Halt – abandon the procedure if there is no descent with three contractions or pulls or if 15 minutes have elapsed.

33.13 CHECKING FOR PROPER APPLICATION OF THE FORCEPS

This helps to prevent injury to the mother and baby.

The *posterior fontanelle* should be located midway between the sides of the blades, with the lambdoid sutures equidistant from the blades and one finger's breadth above the plane of the shanks. A distance greater than this indicates that the head is extended; if the distance is less than one fingerbreadth, this indicates that the head is over-flexed.

The *sagittal suture* must be perpendicular to the plane of the shanks throughout its length.

The *fenestration* of the blades should be barely felt, and the amount of fenestration felt on each side should be equal. If the blades have not been applied deeply enough, the palpable fenestration will be more than a fingertip and the operator is alerted to the risk of facial nerve injury.

33.14 KJELLAND FORCEPS

Key features: slight pelvic curve; overlapping shanks; a sliding lock; knobs that indicate the anterior aspect of the forceps

In direct OP, ROP or LOP position: direct application – same as earlier, but check that the knobs are facing the occiput

In OT position: direct application or wandering method.

! Caution
- Do not perform instrumental delivery unless certain of presentation, the position of the fetal head and cervical dilatation.
- Maternal deaths have been reported from cervical tear when a ventouse cup has been applied before full cervical dilatation.
- The operator must be willing to abandon the procedure if there is no descent of the fetal head.

33.15 TRIAL OF INSTRUMENTAL DELIVERY

When there are features suggesting that vaginal delivery is feasible but could be difficult, a trial of instrumental delivery is acceptable practice, provided that this is performed in theatre with ready recourse to

CS if needed. The features include prolonged labour, one-fifth of the baby's head palpable abdominally, occipito-posterior position, presenting part at the level of the spines, excessive caput, macrosomia and body mass index >30. Selection of cases is important, and a trial of instrumental delivery is inappropriate where there is obstructed labour. A trial in theatre is not a justification for attempting high forceps delivery.

- Inform the consultant before proceeding.
- Inform the anaesthetist and paediatrician.
- Fully explain the plan to the woman and her partner. Obtain consent for CS to be performed if the trial of instrumental delivery fails. Also, keep the couple informed during the procedure.
- There should be CTG monitoring while setting up for anaesthesia/delivery, as well as during the interval between an unsuccessful trial and CS.
- Cord blood analysis (pH and base excess) should be performed.

33.15.1 Decision-making

A trial of instrumental delivery is, as its name suggests, a trial, and proceeding to a CS should not be seen as a failure. There is no room for heroism. If rotation, descent and delivery are not readily accomplished, proceed to CS.

33.16 THE PRINCIPLE OF ABANDONMENT

This applies to presumed straightforward instrumental deliveries and those conducted as a trial in theatre. An attempt at instrumental vaginal delivery should be halted if:

- There is difficulty in applying the instrument.
- There is no descent with each pull.
- Delivery is not imminent following three pulls of a correctly applied instrument.
- 15 minutes (or 20 minutes, depending on the local protocol) has elapsed and the baby has not been delivered.

If any of the above apply:

- The accoucheur should resist the temptation to try one more time.
- A second instrument should not be used.

33.17 POST-DELIVERY

- Ensure that instruments and swabs are accounted for, and document this.
- Administer thromboembolism prophylaxis as appropriate.
- Give analgesia as appropriate.
- Perform a cord blood analysis (pH and base excess).
- Examine the baby for any scalp, facial or other injuries.
- Recommend vitamin K.

- Provide full documentation (see next section).
- If there are any complications, discuss these with the woman.
- Bladder care: observe for urinary retention.

33.18 DOCUMENTATION

The following should be documented:

- Indication
- Anaesthesia
- Instrument(s) used
- Findings on examination: fifths palpable; position and station of the fetal head; degree of moulding and caput; adequacy of pelvis
- Procedure, including ease of application of instrument, number of pulls and number of detachments, if any
- Time of commencement and completion
- Condition of the baby, including findings on examination
- Assessment of the vagina and perineum after delivery
- Findings on rectal examination after delivery
- Any complications and how they were managed
- Swab count
- Cord pH
- Details of perineal repair, if applicable

The use of a proforma (paper or electronic format) incorporating the aforementioned has been shown to improve documentation.

33.19 ERRORS IN INSTRUMENTAL VAGINAL DELIVERY

Table 33.2 shows examples of errors in instrumental vaginal delivery.

TABLE 33.2 Examples of Errors in Instrumental Vaginal Delivery

TYPE OF ERROR	DESCRIPTION	POSSIBLE CONSEQUENCE	SAFE PRACTICE
A: Action			
Action omitted	Abdominal palpation not done	Level of presenting part misjudged	Use of proforma/checklist
Action mistimed	Rotation done during a contraction	Cervical spine injury to the fetus	Rotate only when uterus is relaxed
Action too long or too short	Prolonged traction	Intracranial injury	Stick to time limits and number of pulls
Action in wrong direction	Traction directed forwards and upwards too soon; this causes premature extension of the head as a result of which a larger circumference of the head emerges at the introitus	Third-degree perineal tear	Mind axis of traction
Action excessive	Continuous traction applied	Compression of fetal head	Only apply traction during a contraction
B: Information retrieval			
Information not retrieved	No assessment regarding thromboprophylaxis	Prophylaxis not prescribed	Incorporate this assessment into documentation proforma
	History of diabetes disregarded	Shoulder dystocia not anticipated	Identify background risk factors before offering instrumental delivery
Wrong information retrieved	Mistaken head level or position	Misapplication of instrument; trauma	Double check
	Thinking the cervix is fully dilated when it is not	Cervical tear	
Incomplete information retrieved	Failure to assess moulding	Traumatic delivery; brain injury	Adopt systematic approach to assessment
	Omission of equipment check	Delay in delivery; stress and impairment of cognition	
C: Procedural checks			
Check omitted or not properly done	Failure to ensure cup does not catch tissue	Vaginal laceration	Training
	Check for proper application of forceps not done as described in text	Trauma to baby's face or eye; facial nerve injury	Understand reason for check
	No check for descent with pull	Undue traction applied	Beware of confirmation bias
	PR not done at end of procedure	Third-degree tear missed	Include VE, PR, swab check in documentation
	VE not done at end of procedure	Retained swab in vagina	
	Swabs not counted		

D: Communication

Failure to communicate	With woman With midwife With senior colleague With anaesthetist With paediatrician	Valid consent not obtained Patient given conflicting information Required supervision not provided Inadequate analgesia Neonatal resuscitation delayed	Verbal and eye contact: empathy Preoperative briefing Teamwork

E: Selection (choosing from a number of options)

	Wrong ventouse cup type Ill-advised sequential instrumentation	Avoidable failure of ventouse Neonatal handicap	See text

F: Cognition

Failure to anticipate	Failure to anticipate PPH in prolonged labour	Massive haemorrhage	Have Syntocinon infusion ready at delivery
Failure to ask the right questions	No descent despite traction: is position correctly determined? Is pulling in the right direction?	Trauma	Situational awareness
	Forceps have less than secure grip of head: is there undiagnosed OP? Is forceps applied over baby's face?	Trauma	Situational awareness

Source: Reproduced with permission from Edozien, Leroy C. Towards safe practice in instrumental vaginal delivery. *Best Prac Clin Obstet Gynaecol.* 2007;21:639–55

Trial of vaginal delivery after a previous caesarean section

34

All women with a uterine scar should have been assessed antenatally and a decision made as to mode of delivery (trial of vaginal delivery or elective CS). In those presenting in labour without antenatal assessment, an experienced obstetrician should review the situation and counsel as appropriate.

Success rate: 3 in 4; 8–9 in 10 if the woman previously had a vaginal birth.

Scar rupture risk: One previous CS – 1 in 200; Two or more previous CS – 1 in 50–100

For twin pregnancies, birth outcomes and success rates are similar to a trial of vaginal birth after previous CS in singleton gestations.

34.1 CONTRAINDICATIONS

- Previous classical CS
- Previous uterine rupture
- Placenta praevia
- Previous myomectomy in which the uterine cavity was breached

34.2 ACTION PLAN FOR TRIAL OF VAGINAL DELIVERY

- Inform the woman of the risk of scar rupture (see earlier)
- Obtain IV access
- FBC
- Group-and-save
- Monitor maternal pulse and BP
- Set up continuous electronic fetal monitoring
- Exclude malpresentation
- Offer epidural analgesia

Once labour is established, assess the cervix every 3 hours.

If the woman has not had a vaginal delivery previously, expect her progress to follow the pattern of a primipara.

A repeat of CS is indicated when the alert line on the partogram has been crossed by 2–3 hours.

DOI: 10.1201/9781315099897-40

34.3 USE OF SYNTOCINON

- Syntocinon (oxytocin) should be used only with the approval of a senior obstetrician.
- It is relatively safe in the latent phase of labour, but high-risk if used to augment labour in the active phase.
- The woman must be informed of the increased risk of scar rupture (about 1 in 50–100). This discussion should be documented.
- Scar rupture is more likely to occur if prostaglandin has been given.
- Dose increments should be given at 30-minute intervals.
- Proceed to CS if there is no change in cervical dilatation 2 hours after commencement of Syntocinon infusion despite good uterine action.
- Be extra vigilant for signs of imminent or actual scar rupture (see next): proceed to CS if any sign is observed.

34.4 SIGNS OF SCAR RUPTURE OR IMMINENT RUPTURE

Things to look out for include:

- Abnormal CTG (the most common sign)
- Poor progress in labour
- Sudden cessation of contractions
- Reduction in intensity of contractions
- Maternal tachycardia or hypotension
- Abdominal pain occurring between contractions
- Shoulder tip or chest pain
- Acute onset of tenderness at the CS scar site
- Vaginal bleeding

If rupture is suspected, then proceed to emergency CS.

! Uterine rupture may occur without any warning signs.

34.5 POST-DELIVERY

Transcervical palpation of the lower segment to exclude a scar rupture after vaginal delivery should not be performed routinely. It may be used to exclude a scar rupture if PPH occurs.

Induction of labour

35

The indication for induction and the patient's consent should be documented.

High-risk inductions should be commenced on the delivery suite.

Ideally, the woman would have been offered membrane sweep before admission to the delivery suite and would have been informed that membrane sweeping is not associated with increased risk of infection but may cause discomfort and bleeding.

In women with an unfavourable cervix, induction of labour is associated with a higher failure rate in nulliparous patients and a higher caesarean section rate in nulliparous and parous patients.

35.1 METHODS

- **Intracervical catheter: Foley catheter or Cook silicone double-balloon catheter.**
  - Procedure for Cook balloon.
  - Explanations **and consent**. CTG for at least 20 minutes.
  - Speculum examination and cleansing of the cervix and clean the cervix.
  - Insert the catheter until both balloons are in the cervical canal and inflate the uterine balloon to 40 mL.
  - Pull back until the inflated balloon is resting against the internal os.
  - Inflate the vaginal balloon with 20 mL N/Saline.
  - Remove the speculum and inflate both balloons to 80 mL each, in increments of 20 mL.
  - Catheter removed after 12 hours.
- **Prostaglandin E$_2$ (PGE$_2$, dinoprostone)**: if membranes are intact and the cervix is unfavourable (os closed or score <7) for ARM.
  - **Gel**: see the algorithms in Figures 35.1–35.3.
  - **Tablets (intravaginal)**: dinoprostone 3 mg to posterior fornix every 6–8 hours; maximum dose 6 mg for all women per course.
- **Slow-release vaginal insert** containing 10 mg dinoprostone (Propess):
  - Insert pessary (in retrieval device) high into posterior fornix and remove when cervical ripening adequate. Remove if cervical ripening inadequate after 24 hours (dose not to be repeated).
  - If the fetal membranes rupture with Propess in situ, record a CTG for 30 minutes and observe uterine activity. Leave Propess in place if CTG is normal and if there is no regular uterine activity.
- **ARM**: if the cervix is favourable and membranes are accessible.
- **Syntocinon (oxytocin) infusion**: if membranes are ruptured. If spontaneous rupture has not occurred, ARM should be performed before commencement of Syntocinon.

DOI: 10.1201/9781315099897-41

Syntocinon infusion should not be started within 6 hours of the last dose of prostaglandin or less than 30 minutes after removal of Propess.

For all methods:

- Confirm indication and gestational age; obtain consent
- Exclude contraindications:
  - Major placenta praevia
  - Abnormal lie
- Commence CTG; if it is abnormal then inform the registrar
- Perform cervical assessment:
  - Cervical score (Table 35.1)
  - Exclude cord presentation
  - Proceed to ARM or prostaglandin induction

35.2 ARTIFICIAL RUPTURE OF FETAL MEMBRANES

The midwife may perform ARM if the following criteria are met:

- The head is engaged
- The vertex is presenting
- Cord presentation has been excluded

Contraindications to ARM are:

- Abnormal lie
- Cord presentation
- Placenta praevia

After ARM, check for cord prolapse and meconium staining of amniotic fluid. Document the fetal heart rate.

TABLE 35.1 Cervical Score

	SCORE			
	0	1	2	3
Dilatation (cm)	<1	1–2	2–4	>4
Length (cm)	>4	2–4	1–2	<1
Consistency	Firm	Average	Soft	
Position	Posterior	Central	Anterior	
Station	-3	-2	-1 or 0	Below spines

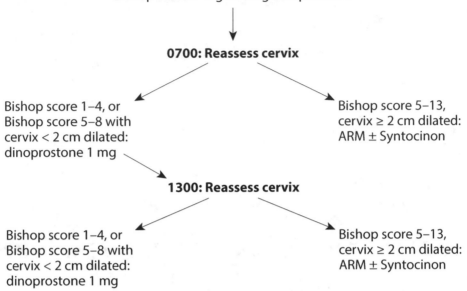

1800–2000: Assess cervix

Bishop score ≤ 4: give 2mg dinoprostone
Bishop score > 4: give 1mg dinoprostone

0700: Reassess cervix

Bishop score 1–4, or
Bishop score 5–8 with
cervix < 2 cm dilated:
dinoprostone 1 mg

Bishop score 5–13,
cervix ≥ 2 cm dilated:
ARM ± Syntocinon

1300: Reassess cervix

Bishop score 1–4, or
Bishop score 5–8 with
cervix < 2 cm dilated:
dinoprostone 1 mg

Bishop score 5–13,
cervix ≥ 2 cm dilated:
ARM ± Syntocinon

If not in labour after three doses dinoprostone, discuss with consultant

FIGURE 35.1   Algorithm for cervical ripening: nullipara.

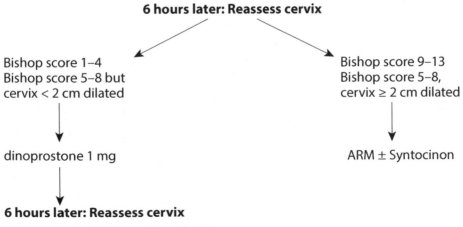

0800–1000: Assess cervix

Bishop score 1–4:
• 2 mg dinoprostone
• if grandmultiparous, 1 mg dinoprostone

Bishop score 5–8 and cervix > 2 cm dilated:
• dinoprostone 1 mg

6 hours later: Reassess cervix

Bishop score 1–4
Bishop score 5–8 but
cervix < 2 cm dilated

Bishop score 9–13
Bishop score 5–8,
cervix ≥ 2 cm dilated

dinoprostone 1 mg

ARM ± Syntocinon

6 hours later: Reassess cervix

• ARM ± Syntocinon, if favourable
• discuss with consultant if unfavourable

FIGURE 35.2   Algorithm for cervical ripening: multipara.

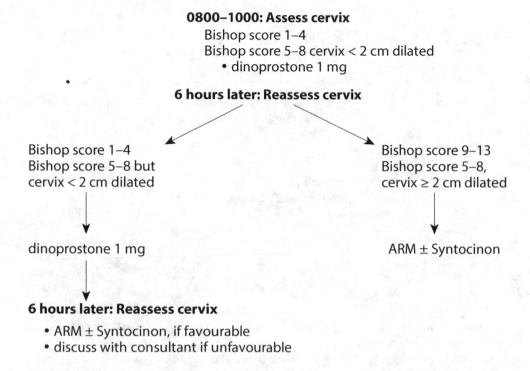

0800–1000: Assess cervix
Bishop score 1–4
Bishop score 5–8 cervix < 2 cm dilated
• dinoprostone 1 mg

6 hours later: Reassess cervix

Bishop score 1–4
Bishop score 5–8 but
cervix < 2 cm dilated

Bishop score 9–13
Bishop score 5–8,
cervix ≥ 2 cm dilated

dinoprostone 1 mg

ARM ± Syntocinon

6 hours later: Reassess cervix

• ARM ± Syntocinon, if favourable
• discuss with consultant if unfavourable

FIGURE 35.3   Algorithm for cervical ripening: previous caesarean section.

35.3 PROSTAGLANDIN INDUCTION OF LABOUR

Use prostaglandin with caution in the following cases:

• Previous CS
• Multiple pregnancy
• Breech presentation
• Compromised fetus (IUGR, oligohydramnios, or abnormal CTG, Doppler ultrasound or bio-physical profile)
• Previous difficult labour or delivery
• Grandmultiparity
• Asthma or glaucoma

35.4 MONITORING FOLLOWING INSERTION OF PROSTAGLANDIN

- CTG monitoring: if normal, discontinue after 1 hour but continue intermittent auscultation.
  - Resume electronic fetal monitoring if any of the following occurs:
  - Contractions commence
  - Vaginal bleeding
  - Rupture of membranes
  - The woman complains of abdominal or back pain
- Maternal pulse, BP and contractions should be monitored half-hourly.
- The woman should remain in bed for 1 hour after administration of prostaglandin.

35.5 PRECAUTIONS

- KY Jelly or chlorhexidine cream should not be used during administration of prostaglandin, since these delay absorption.
- Do not insert prostaglandin if you are unable to feel the cervix.
- Syntocinon should not be started within 6 hours of administering prostaglandin.

35.6 HYPERSTIMULATION

In cases of uterine hyperstimulation, administer tocolysis (see later).

35.7 SYNTOCINON INFUSION

The ideal dosing regimen of oxytocin is not well established. The regime outlined next is an optimal low-dose regime that begins with 2 milliunits/min.

35.7.1 Syntocinon infusion rates should be recorded in mU/min rather than mL/hr

Mix 10 units of Syntocinon in 500 mL compound sodium lactate (Hartmann's solution) or 0.9% saline, which gives a concentration of 20 milliunits/mL; with this dose, an infusion rate of 3 mL/h is equivalent to 1 milliunit/min.

   Commence infusion at 2 milliunits/min (i.e. 6 mL/h); increase every 30 minutes until strong, regular uterine contractions – three in 10 minutes – are obtained.

A syringe driver or infusion pump must be used.

Do not exceed 32 milliunits/min (i.e. 96 mL/h); see Table 15.1.

Do not infuse through the same line as blood, plasma or insulin.

The syringe must be labelled, with the dose of drug and signatures of staff responsible on the label.

If labour is not established after 5 hours on this regimen, then induction should be discontinued.

All women for whom labour is being induced with Syntocinon should have continuous electronic fetal monitoring.

A fluid balance chart should be kept.

The use of Syntocinon in the following circumstances requires the explicit approval of the consultant:

- Multiple pregnancy
- Malpresentation
- Previous CS or other uterine scar
- Grandmultiparity

35.8 UTERINE HYPERSTIMULATION

This can occur with prostaglandin or Syntocinon.

35.8.1 Definition

- More than five contractions per 10-minute interval for at least 20 minutes (uterine tachysystole), or each uterine contraction lasting at least 2 minutes, or increased baseline uterine tone (uterine hypertonus).
- Suspicious or pathological CTG.

35.8.2 Management

- Discontinue Syntocinon infusion.
- Lay the woman on her left side.
- Institute a rapid infusion of 1000 mL 0.9% saline.
- In extreme cases, consider tocolysis with terbutaline 0.25 mg SC. *Note*: This is an off-licence use of terbutaline.
- It may be necessary to deliver the baby – is the CTG back to normal?
- Caution should be exercised in using terbutaline (a betamimetic). It is contraindicated in cardiac diseases.

Antenatal corticosteroid therapy

36

36.1 INDICATIONS

Corticosteroids should be given to women between 24 and 34 completed weeks' gestation presenting with any of the following:

- Threatened preterm delivery
- APH
- Preterm PROM
- Any condition requiring elective preterm delivery

Corticosteroids should be given even if birth is expected within 24 hours, as there will be benefit to the baby.

They are most beneficial in births that occur between 24 hours and 7 days of administration of the second dose.

Cervical length and fetal fibronectin should be used to predict the likelihood of early delivery, to minimize unnecessary antenatal corticosteroid therapy.

36.2 DOSE

Betamethasone 12 mg IM, two doses given 24 hours apart. (If delivery is likely to occur within 24 hours, the second dose may be given after 12 hours.)

Alternative: Dexamethasone 6 mg IM, four doses given 12 hours apart.

36.3 CONTRAINDICATIONS

Corticosteroids should not be given if there are any of the following:

- Clinical evidence of chorioamnionitis
- Uncontrolled diabetes mellitus (see Chapter 53)
- Tuberculosis
- Porphyria

DOI: 10.1201/9781315099897-42

36.4 BETA-SYMPATHOMIMETICS

The combination of steroids and a beta-sympathomimetic tocolytic poses a risk of pulmonary oedema. When this combination is used, IV fluids should be kept to a minimum and a strict fluid balance should be kept. Observe the woman for chest pain, dyspnoea and cough, and discontinue the tocolytic therapy if any of these occur. Blood glucose and U/E should be checked every 6 hours.

36.5 REPEATED DOSES

Excessive prenatal glucocorticoid exposure may be associated with child neurodevelopment consequences as well as cardiovascular and other physiological dysfunction in the adult life, so caution must be exercised with antenatal corticosteroid therapy.

A single repeat course of antenatal corticosteroids should be considered in women who are less than 34 weeks of gestation who are at risk of preterm delivery within 72 hours, and whose prior course of antenatal corticosteroids was administered more than 7 days previously.

Consider the possibility of adrenal insufficiency if a woman or baby who has been exposed to repeated doses of antenatal corticosteroids has an unexplained collapse.

Preterm prelabour rupture of membranes

37

This is the loss of amniotic fluid from the vagina before 37 weeks in the absence of uterine contractions. For management of PROM at term, see Chapter 11.

37.1 ACTION PLAN

37.1.1 If a woman presents with a history suggestive of ruptured membranes

- Perform a sterile speculum examination to confirm the diagnosis and exclude a prolapsed cord. Digital examination is not required unless the woman is in labour.
- Take swabs from the vagina (bacteriology) and endocervix (*Chlamydia*).
- If no amniotic fluid seen, test vaginal fluid for insulin-like growth factor-binding protein 1 (IGFBP-1) or placental alpha microglobulin-1 (PAMG-1). The detection of PAMG-1 or elevated IGFBP-1 is a marker for preterm labour.

If test result is positive, manage as clinically indicated.
If test result is negative and no other concerns, discharge home.

- FBC and group-and-save.
- Obtain a midstream specimen of urine.
- Perform an ultrasound scan for presentation, fetal growth and amniotic fluid volume.
- Liaise with the paediatrician.
- If in established labour (or delivery within 24 hours planned) at <30 weeks of gestation, offer intravenous magnesium sulphate for neuroprotection of the baby.
- Offer psychological support to woman and partner.

Conservative management is indicated if infection is excluded and the woman is not in labour.
Delivery is indicated if any of the following occur:

- Maternal pyrexia
- Fetal tachycardia
- Uterine tenderness
- Meconium staining of amniotic fluid
- Elevated CRP and/or leukocytosis (note that steroids may elevate the white cell count)

DOI: 10.1201/9781315099897-43

- Offensive amniotic fluid
- Gestation reaches 37 weeks

37.2 CONSERVATIVE MANAGEMENT

- Alert the neonatal unit.
- Give antibiotics after initial vaginal examination:
  - Erythromycin 250 mg four times a day for 10 days or until the woman is in established labour, whichever is sooner.
  If she cannot tolerate erythromycin or erythromycin is contraindicated, offer an oral penicillin for a maximum of 10 days or until she is in established labour, whichever is sooner.
  - **Do not give co-amoxiclav**, since this is associated with an increased risk of necrotizing enterocolitis in the newborn.
- Give betamethasone 12 mg IM, two doses 24 hours apart if gestation <34 weeks.
- Take temperature and pulse rate 4-hourly.
- Monitor fetal heart rate daily.
- FBC and CRP twice weekly.
- Perform an ultrasound/Doppler scan weekly (for amniotic fluid volume and fetal breathing movement).
- Scan fortnightly for fetal growth.

Continue to 37 weeks if no contraindication.

37.3 MODE OF DELIVERY, IN THE ABSENCE OF OTHER COMPLICATIONS

- Cephalic presentation: vaginal delivery.
- Breech presentation: discuss with the woman and her partner the risks and benefits of CS versus vaginal delivery.

37.4 INDUCTION OF LABOUR

- Syntocinon (oxytocin) infusion: see Table 15.1 for regimen.
- Prostaglandin may be used to ripen an unfavourable cervix and induce labour after preterm PROM, but:
  - Insert during a sterile vaginal examination
  - Use only one dose

37.5 LABOUR

- Continue monitoring for signs of infection (temperature and pulse).
- Inform the paediatrician.
- Screen the baby for sepsis.

Preterm uterine contractions

38

38.1 DIAGNOSIS

- Regular contractions (at least one every 10 minutes).
- Progressive cervical effacement and/or dilatation.
- Less than 37 completed weeks of gestation.

38.2 ACTION PLAN

- Confirm gestational age
- Assess for symptoms of urinary tract infection
- Assess for physical or emotional trauma
- Check temperature and pulse
- Check for uterine tenderness (consider placental abruption and chorioamnionitis)
- Assess frequency and duration of contractions
- Assess fetal lie, presentation and station
- If gestational age ≥30 weeks, consider transvaginal ultrasound measurement of cervical length
  If cervical length >15 mm, preterm labour unlikely
- Perform a speculum examination
- Exclude rupture of membranes
- If gestational age ≥30 weeks and cervical length scan not feasible, offer fetal fibronectin test. If concentration ≤50 ng/mL, preterm labour is unlikely
- Vaginal swab and endocervical swab
- Assess the cervix
- Obtain a midstream specimen of urine
- FBC
- U/E
- Perform a Kleihauer test if the mother is Rh-negative
- CTG
- If there are <34 completed weeks, give corticosteroid: betamethasone 12 mg IM, two doses 24 hours apart. **Steroids should not be used if there is clinical chorioamnionitis and should be used with caution in women with diabetes**
- Inform the consultant obstetrician
- Determine the underlying cause if possible
- Consider transfer to a tertiary centre
- Decide (with the consultant) which of the following management options is to be followed:
  - Suppression of labour (but see the contraindications later)

DOI: 10.1201/9781315099897-44

- Allow progression to vaginal delivery (see later)
- CS, if indicated
- Observation, if the diagnosis of preterm labour is uncertain
- Discuss with the parents regarding prognosis and management
- Inform the paediatrician and neonatal unit

38.3 FETAL FIBRONECTIN TEST

38.3.1 Indications

- Contractile uterine activity between $22+0$ and $36+0$ weeks gestation
- Intact membranes
- Cervical dilatation $\leq$3cm

38.3.2 Contraindications

- Ruptured membranes
- Cervical suture in place
- Cervical dilation >3 cm
- Presence of soaps, gels, lubricants or disinfectants

38.3.3 Relative contraindications

- Bleeding
- Within 24 hours of coitus (Coitus may cause a false positive result, as might digital examination and transvaginal ultrasound scan)

38.3.4 Procedure

- Examine using a sterile speculum.
- Use only sterile water (as other lubricants or disinfectant may cause a false negative result).
- Obtain sample for testing from the posterior fornix of the vagina.

If fFN <50 ng/mL (negative), the risk of birth within 7–14 days is low.

38.4 MANAGEMENT OF ESTABLISHED PRETERM LABOUR (WHEN IT IS TOO LATE TO SUPPRESS LABOUR)

- Institute continuous electronic fetal monitoring.
- Avoid narcotic analgesia.
- Avoid FBS if <34 weeks.

- Avoid vacuum-assisted if <34 weeks.
- Alert paediatrician/SCBU (paediatric team to be present at delivery).
- Episiotomy is indicated if there is delay due to the head pushing against a tight perineum.
- Do not use 'prophylactic' forceps.

See also management of the pre-viable fetus (Chapter 39) and management of preterm breech presentation (Chapter 44).

There is no evidence to justify the routine use of prophylactic antibiotics for preterm labour with intact membranes.

38.5 SUPPRESSION OF LABOUR

38.5.1 Aims

- To enable the use of steroids for accelerating lung maturity.
- To allow in utero transfer, if necessary.

38.5.2 Options

- Nifedipine (unlicensed for use in preterm labour)
- Indomethacin (unlicensed)
- Atosiban (licensed)

Nifedipine is effective in suppressing preterm labour and has fewer side effects and better neonatal outcome (lower incidence of jaundice, RDS and intraventricular haemorrhage).

Indomethacin is also effective but is associated with premature closure of the fetal ductus arteriosus. This is more common in fetuses >32 weeks and where indomethacin has been administered for >48 hours.

Atosiban has significantly fewer maternal and fetal adverse effects. However, it is substantially more expensive.

! A pragmatic approach is to use nifedipine or indomethacin initially. If the response is inadequate, then a combination of both may be used. If response remains poor, or if contractions recur, then use atosiban.

38.6 CONTRAINDICATIONS TO SUPPRESSION OF LABOUR

Do not attempt to suppress labour if any of the following apply:

- Gestational age >35 weeks
- Cervix >4 cm dilated

- Signs/symptoms of chorioamnionitis
- Abnormal CTG
- IUGR
- Placental abruption
- Bleeding (other than spotting) from placenta praevia
- Hypertension/pre-eclampsia
- Maternal thyroid or cardiac disease
- Intrauterine fetal death
- Fetal abnormality not compatible with survival

! Before administering a tocolytic, exclude medical contraindications to the drug.

38.7 NIFEDIPINE

Note: Do not use with magnesium sulphate or in women with significant cardiac disease.

As the use of nifedipine for preterm labour is off-label, it should be used strictly according to the local protocol.

Contraindicated in women with cardiac disease or hypotension.

If necessary, preload with 500 mL compound sodium lactate (Hartmann's solution) – because nifedipine is a calcium channel blocker and therefore lowers BP.

Its tocolytic effect starts at 30–60 minutes after administration.

38.7.1 Loading dose

Oral: (crush or chew to enhance absorption) 20 mg stat; repeat after 30 minutes if contractions persist. If contractions have not ceased by 3 hours, consider a second line tocolytic.

Alternatively, 10 mg sublingually (the woman bites into the capsule and holds the liquid under her tongue). Repeat every 15 minutes until uterine contractions cease, up to a maximum dose of 40 mg (four capsules).

Maximum daily dose of Nifedipine immediate release: 160 mg/day

38.7.2 Maintenance dose

20 mg tds for 72 hours

- This is commenced 6 hours after the loading dose.
- Side effects: headache, palpitations, nausea, tachycardia.

38.8 INDOMETHACIN (PROSTAGLANDINS SYNTHETASE INHIBITOR)

Give 100 mg rectally as an initial dose, followed by 50 mg orally every 6 hours for 48 hours.

If regular uterine contractions persist 2 hours after the initial dose, an additional 100 mg suppository is administered before beginning oral therapy.

Avoid the use indomethacin if the gestational age >32 weeks (prolonged use may cause premature closure of the ductus arteriosus) or if there is maternal or fetal renal disease or severe oligohydramnios. If therapy continues beyond 48 hours (unlikely), scan for amniotic fluid volume (it could cause oligohydramnios as a result of reduced renal blood flow). Indomethacin is also contraindicated where there is a history of peptic ulcers or allergies to NSAIDs. It inhibits platelet aggregation, so it should be used with caution in cases of APH or bleeding problems.

Side effects: (rare) headache.

38.9 ATOSIBAN

38.9.1 Loading bolus

Give 6.75 mg IV as a bolus over 1 minute:

- Take a vial of atosiban 7.5 mg/mL and draw 0.9 mL; this contains the required loading dose of 6.75 mg.
    Loading infusion Give 18 mg/h (300 µg/min) IV for 3 hours.
    Maintenance dose Give 6 mg/h (100 µg/min) IV for 3–45 hours.
- Take two 5 mL vials each containing atosiban 7.5 mg/mL concentrate. Withdraw 10 mL from a 100 mL bag of 0.9% saline, leaving 90 mL. Add the contents of the atosiban vials to the 90 mL saline. This gives a solution of atosiban 75 mg/100 mL. Infuse this at 24 mL/h for 3 hours (loading infusion), then reduce to 8 mL/h maintenance infusion).

The infusion is discontinued about 6 hours after contractions have ceased. The duration of treatment should not exceed 48 hours.

TABLE 38.1   Regimen for Atosiban Infusion

STEP	REGIMEN	INFUSION RATE	ATOSIBAN DOSE
1	0.9 mL intravenous bolus injection given over 1 minute	Not applicable	6.75 mg
2	3 hours intravenous loading infusion	24 mL/hour (300 µg/min)	54 mg
3	Up to 45 hours subsequent intravenous infusion	8 mL/hour (100 µg/min)	Up to 270 mg

The total dose given during a full course of atosiban therapy should preferably not exceed 330.75 mg of atosiban.

Side effects include nausea, vomiting, headache and tachycardia.

38.10 MAGNESIUM SULPHATE FOR NEUROPROTECTION

Indicated in GA 23^{+0}–33^{+6}

4 g intravenous bolus of magnesium sulphate over 15 minutes, followed by an intravenous infusion of 1 g per hour until the birth or for 24 hours (whichever is sooner)

Monitor the following at least every 4 hours, to elicit signs of toxicity: pulse, blood pressure, respiratory rate and deep tendon reflexes.

38.11 MONITORING

Women on tocolytic drugs should be closely monitored:

- CTG
- Frequency and strength of contractions
- Side effects of medication

Clinical judgement should determine whether further cervical assessment is required following administration of a tocolytic. Unnecessary vaginal examination should be avoided.

Deliveries at the lower margin of viability

39

39.1 PREGNANCY UNDER 22 WEEKS

- The following points should be discussed and documented.
- Only 1 in 100 babies will survive and, of these, half will have a severe disability.
- Delivery may be rapid.
- The baby may be born alive, move and/or gasp.
- Document the agreed management plan in the case notes.

Regardless of gestational age, if a baby shows any sign of life after delivery but subsequently dies, it should be registered as a live birth and neonatal death.

39.2 PREGNANCY OVER 22 WEEKS

- The following points should be discussed and documented.
- The baby may survive short-term.
- Delivery may be rapid.
- A paediatrician and the SCBU must be informed.
- Give the parents an information leaflet about the very premature baby.
- Document the agreed management plan in the case notes.

A paediatrician should attend any birth after 20 weeks' gestation, because:

- The baby may be born alive.
- There may have been an error in assessment of gestational age.
- A decision not to resuscitate should be made by a paediatrician, not by an obstetrician or midwife.

! If the woman wishes to use the toilet, the midwife should be alert. It is not uncommon for the small baby to be delivered in the toilet.

DOI: 10.1201/9781315099897-45

39.3 POST-DELIVERY CARE IF THE BABY DOES NOT SURVIVE

- Inform the consultant obstetrician of the birth.
- Agree postnatal care according to the wishes of the parents, and inform the GP, consultant obstetrician and community midwife.
- Inform the antenatal clinic and parent education coordinator.
- Offer post-delivery support, e.g. a link with the support group (see next section).
- Inform the woman of the potential benefits of the recommended tests and investigations, and instigate as appropriate.
- Offer keepsakes and photographs.
- Discuss funeral arrangements and issue necessary documentation.
- Offer the opportunity to take the baby home before the funeral and make necessary arrangements with the funeral director.

! All live births must be registered, regardless of gestational age.

39.4 SUPPORT GROUP

Sands (Stillbirth & Neonatal Death Charity)
Sands Helpline
t: 0808 164 3332
e: helpline@sands.org.uk
General enquiries 020 7436 7940/020 3897 6094
Website: www.sands.org.uk/

Multiple pregnancy

40

Triplets and higher-order pregnancies are normally delivered by elective CS. If the woman presents with uterine contractions, then the consultant should be informed immediately and a decision will be taken regarding the timing of delivery, depending on the frequency and strength of contractions. If the woman is in established labour, then arrangements should be started for an urgent CS.

The following guidelines apply to the management of **twin pregnancies**.

40.1 FIRST STAGE OF LABOUR

- The plan of management should be stated clearly antenatally; look for the plan in the case notes.
- On admission in labour:
  - Inform the registrar and anaesthetist.
  - Secure IV access.
  - FBC and group-and-save.
  - Set up continuous electronic monitoring of both twins (dual monitor).
  - Recommend epidural analgesia.
- Examine lie/presentation of both twins, with the aid of an ultrasound scan:
  - **If both twins are cephalic**, proceed as with normal vaginal delivery.
  - **If the first twin is cephalic and the second twin non-cephalic**, anticipate normal delivery of the first twin, with possible recourse to CS if there are problems with the second twin.
  - **If the first twin is non-cephalic**, recommend CS.
- Prepare two neonatal resuscitation units.

! Ensure that the CTG monitor is recording the heart rates of both twins, not a duplication of one twin's heart rate – be suspicious if the two traces are identical (or appear to be). Where there is doubt, application of a scalp electrode to the leading twin may be helpful.

Syntocinon (oxytocin) may be used to augment contractions, but this must be discussed first with a senior obstetrician.

Possible scenarios in the second stage should be discussed early in labour, so that the mother can prepare her mind for what may happen, e.g. delivery in theatre and manoeuvres to deliver the second twin. This is particularly important if the presentation of the second twin is non-cephalic, since the risk of having a CS after normal delivery of the first twin is (in the author's own experience) approximately 1 in 9. If the presentation of the second twin is non-cephalic, then delivery should be conducted in theatre; alternatively, it could be conducted in an adjacent room, with regional anaesthesia and the theatre team primed.

DOI: 10.1201/9781315099897-46

40.2 SECOND STAGE OF LABOUR

- The following should be present: an experienced obstetrician, a paediatrician, two midwives and an anaesthetist.
- While the leading twin is being delivered, an assistant should attempt to stabilize the lie of the second twin.
- Record the time of delivery of the first twin. **Do not give Syntometrine** (ergometrine with oxytocin).
- Ensure that the umbilical cord is clamped properly (this is important in the case of shared fetal circulation). Use an additional clamp or marked clamps to distinguish the cords of the twins.
- Confirm the lie and presentation of the second twin by ultrasound scan.
- Perform a pelvic examination to assess presentation and descent.

40.3 DELIVERY OF THE SECOND TWIN

Continue CTG monitoring. As long as the trace is normal, there is no reason to be worried about the clock, but CTG abnormalities are common when 30 minutes have elapsed.

40.3.1 Cephalic presentation

Confirm that the presenting part is in the pelvis. It will commonly be necessary to hold the baby's head over the pelvic brim. Perform ARM with the next uterine contraction, taking care to exclude cord presentation.

If there is a delay in re-establishing uterine contractions, start Syntocinon infusion: 10 units in 500 mL 0.9% saline or compound sodium lactate (Hartmann's solution); commence at 6 mL/h and double the rate every 5 minutes.

If uncomplicated vertex delivery is imminent, the midwife can deliver.

40.3.2 Breech presentation

- Offer ECV. If ECV is accepted and is successful, then proceed as described earlier for cephalic presentation. If a Syntocinon infusion is running, it should be discontinued to facilitate ECV. It may be necessary to relax the uterus with IV glyceryl trinitrate or SC terbutaline.
- If ECV is declined or is attempted unsuccessfully, then assisted breech delivery should be conducted by the obstetrician or a midwife skilled in the conduct of breech delivery.
- Before rupturing the membranes, ensure that the presenting part is in the pelvis – it will usually be necessary to hold the breech over the pelvic brim.

- Where ECV and assisted breech delivery are both declined, CS will have to be performed.
- In cases of footling breech, the options are breech extraction and CS.

40.3.3 Lie not longitudinal

The options are:

- Internal podalic version: grasp a foot vaginally through intact membranes, pull it down gently, and then perform ARM. An assisted breech delivery is then accomplished. This should always be performed in theatre.
- ECV, then proceed as described earlier for cephalic presentation.

If the prior options fail, or in the absence of an obstetrician skilled in podalic version, then resort to CS rather than try anything heroic.

40.3.4 Internal podalic version and breech extraction

The indications are:

- Transverse lie
- Failed ECV
- Fetal distress

Do not attempt this if the membranes have ruptured.

The uterus should be well relaxed; do not perform during a contraction, and discontinue Syntocinon infusion if one has been running. If necessary, IV glyceryl trinitrate (100 µg repeated at 2-minute intervals) or SC terbutaline 0.25 mg may be given to relax the uterus.

Preferably both feet of the baby should be grasped if breech extraction rather than assisted breech delivery is intended. If only one foot can be reached, this should be the anterior foot; if the posterior foot has been grasped, it should be rotated 180° to make it anterior – this is to avoid having the anterior buttock wedged astride the symphysis pubes.

Beware not to pull down an arm instead of the legs. The heel distinguishes a foot from a hand. Do not bring down a foot until the heel has been identified.

> 'I cannot emphasise too strongly that there is a world of difference between assisted breech delivery and breech extraction. The first necessitates only a series of simple manipulations with minimal analgesic or anaesthetic requirements. The second is – or can be – a formidable operation, with considerable danger to the fetus, and one which requires the help of full anaesthesia or major nerve-blocking procedures. Many a fetus is lost because an inexperienced medical attendant plunges into the second line of treatment when the conditions and preparations are suitable only for the first.'
>
> Myerscough PR. *Munro Kerr's Operative Obstetrics*, 10th edn. London: Baillière Tindall, 1982:76

40.4 THIRD STAGE OF LABOUR

- Active management should be used in the third stage – physiological management is contraindicated.
- Administer a Syntocinon infusion, 40 units in 500 mL for 4 hours.
- Perform a full examination of the placenta and membranes.
- If the twins are of the same sex, send the placenta for histological examination (to confirm chorionicity).

40.5 INDICATIONS FOR CS FOR SECOND TWIN

- Acute fetal distress with vaginal delivery not imminent.
- Failure of the second twin to descend into the pelvis.
- Transverse lie with failed external version.
- Maternal haemorrhage, with vaginal delivery not imminent.
- Obstetrician not skilled in internal podalic version or breech extraction.

Abnormal lie in labour

41

This can be transverse or oblique.

- Exclude placenta praevia, ovarian cyst, uterine fibroids and other possible causes
- CTG
- Inform the woman of the risk of cord prolapse
- Vaginal examination:
  - Exclude cord presentation
  - Assess the cervix
  - Exclude ruptured membranes

41.1 INTACT MEMBRANES

- If there are no contraindications, then discuss ECV (see Chapter 45).
- If ECV is declined or is attempted unsuccessfully, then proceed to CS.
- Following successful version, consider ARM (in theatre) plus Syntocinon (oxytocin).

41.2 RUPTURED MEMBRANES

- Avoid external version
- Exclude arm prolapse
- Deliver by CS

41.3 CAESAREAN SECTION

Obtain consent for 'caesarean section', not 'lower-segment caesarean section'.
Check before the operation whether the fetal back is inferior or superior:

- If the back is superior then it is easy to reach for the baby's legs and proceed with breech delivery, but beware that an arm may protrude from the uterine incision (put it back) or may be mistaken for a foot (look for the heel).
- If the back is inferior then internal version will usually be required, and the breech is usually easier to bring down than the head.

DOI: 10.1201/9781315099897-47

41.4 DIFFICULT CASES

For a preterm baby with the back inferior, a low vertical uterine incision should be considered.

For transverse lie with arm prolapse, a classical CS should be considered. If a transverse incision is used, then this will almost always be converted to a J-incision and/or the baby will suffer a traumatic delivery. If a transverse incision is used then additional measures – such as relaxing or distending the uterus – should be employed (see next).

In some cases, it may be necessary to relax the uterus to facilitate delivery of the baby. This can be achieved with SC terbutaline 0.25 µg or IV glyceryl trinitrate 100 µg.

41.5 UTERODISTENSION

For difficult cases **where the fetal membranes have ruptured**, the author devised the technique of utero-distension to facilitate lower-segment CS delivery. These cases include transverse lie with arm prolapse and early preterm delivery with longitudinal lie and ruptured membranes, where a classical incision would otherwise be indicated.

In this technique, 500–1000 mL of warm (room temperature) 0.9% saline is infused via a giving set inserted into the uterine cavity through a stab (1.0 cm) incision in the lower pole of the uterus. Pressure on the bag of fluid is required. Once the cavity is sufficiently distended, the incision is extended and the baby is delivered. This technique allows the use of a low incision where a classical (upper segment) incision would otherwise have been necessary.

Occipito-posterior position

42

This should be suspected if:

- The baby's back is difficult to feel.
- Fetal heart tones are heard better towards the flank.
- There is significant back pain.

Confirm by vaginal examination.

To ensure rotation of the head, good uterine activity is required, so consider the use of Syntocinon (oxytocin) if the frequency and strength of contractions are suboptimal, particularly in a nulliparous woman. This also reduces the chances of a prolonged labour.

Hands-and-knees maternal posture may influence fetal position.

42.1 PERSISTENT OCCIPITO-POSTERIOR POSITION

The options for effecting vaginal delivery are:

- Vacuum-assisted delivery, with posterior cup
- Kjelland forceps delivery
- Manual rotation:
  - Lithotomy position (or left lateral)
  - Adequate analgesia

Ensure that the criteria for instrumental delivery are met before proceeding with forceps or ventouse.

Nulliparity and occipito-posterior position carry a high risk of injury to the anal sphincter complex, so an episiotomy is recommended.

In skilled hands, the Kiwi OmniCup vacuum device is as good as Kjelland forceps in effecting rotation, as well as less traumatic to the mother.

DOI: 10.1201/9781315099897-48

Malpresentation

43

The baby's presentation reflects the degree of flexion or extension of the head:

- Full flexion: occiput
- Full extension: face
- Deflexed but not fully extended: brow

- Inform the registrar or senior obstetrician
- Group-and-save
- Rule out fetal abnormalities (anencephaly, goitre and hydocephalus)

43.1 BROW PRESENTATION

The forehead is the presenting part palpable on vaginal examination. Frontal sutures, anterior fontanelle, orbital ridges, eyes and the root of the nose are palpable.

This may change to a face or vertex presentation, and so, if the woman is in early labour, await events. If there is slow progress or secondary arrest, proceed to CS. If diagnosed in advanced labour, then CS is indicated.

43.2 FACE PRESENTATION

This is diagnosed by palpation of the chin, mouth, nose and orbital ridges. It may be mistaken for a breech presentation.

If the woman is in early labour and cephalo-pelvic disproportion has been excluded, allow to progress.
If the woman is in advanced labour, check whether the position is mentoanterior or mentoposterior:

- If it is mentoanterior, then vaginal delivery is feasible; allow to progress, proceeding to CS if progress is poor. An episiotomy will usually be required.
- If it is mentoposterior, then vaginal delivery is not feasible, but there is a 1 in 4 chance of rotation on reaching the pelvic floor, so you may wait and see; if the position is persistently mentoposterior then perform CS.

Where vaginal delivery is anticipated, inform the mother in advance that the baby's face may be temporarily swollen (oedema) and this may cause initial difficulties with feeding.
If there are CTG abnormalities, then proceed to CS. Note that FBS is contraindicated.
At CS, flex and rotate the head to occipito-transverse before delivery.

DOI: 10.1201/9781315099897-49

43.3 COMPOUND PRESENTATION

This could be a cephalic presentation with a foot or hand palpable or a breech presentation with a hand palpable (take care to distinguish between hand and foot).

Manage as normal for a cephalic or breech presentation, unless there is cord prolapse.

Breech presentation

44

Breech presentation may be diagnosed antenatally or in labour.

For cases of persistent breech presentation (including after ECV) diagnosed antenatally, the mode of delivery should be stated clearly in the antenatal records. This should be either a planned CS or a *planned vaginal birth*.

Suggested criteria for planned vaginal birth:

- A skilled attendant is available.
- Hyperextended neck on ultrasound excluded.
- Estimated fetal weight <3.5 kg.
- Footling presentation excluded.
- No fetal distress or growth restriction.

44.1 UNDIAGNOSED BREECH IN LABOUR

- Confirm the presentation by ultrasound scan.
- Determine the wishes of the mother regarding mode of delivery.
- If the membranes are intact, assess suitability for ECV (see Chapter 45).
- Recommend CS if any of the following occur:
  - Pelvis clinically small or anatomically abnormal
  - Placenta praevia
  - Big baby (consider parity and the weight of previous babies delivered vaginally)
  - Hyperextended fetal head
  - Footling presentation
  - IUGR
  - Previous perinatal death
  - Bad obstetric history
  - Medical problems or other risk factors
- The mode of delivery should always be discussed with the consultant.

44.2 PRETERM BREECH IN LABOUR

- Inform the consultant.
- Offer epidural analgesia (which prevents pushing before full cervical dilatation).

DOI: 10.1201/9781315099897-50

There is insufficient evidence to justify routine CS for preterm breech. The decision regarding mode of delivery should be made after full discussion with the woman (and her partner, if present). The discussion should be documented.

44.3 BREECH VAGINAL DELIVERY

44.3.1 First stage of labour

- Discuss the risks of breech vaginal delivery.
- Discuss epidural analgesia (which prevents pushing before full cervical dilatation and facilitates delivery, but may inhibit pushing in the second stage).
- Institute continuous electronic fetal monitoring. A monitoring electrode may be applied to the buttock if an abdominal transducer is not giving a good trace.
- Obtain IV access: FBC and group-and-save.
- The anaesthetist must be available immediately.
- Alert the paediatrician.
- Explain the delivery to the woman and partner/relative (involving the latter is important, since they will observe the delivery).
- ARM is performed only if the presenting part is applied well to the cervix.
- Perform a vaginal examination immediately after spontaneous rupture of membranes (to exclude cord prolapse).
- Following spontaneous or artificial rupture of membranes, observe the CTG closely for the first 10 minutes (because of the risk of occult cord prolapse).
- Give oral ranitidine 150 mg.
- Poor progress despite good contractions suggests that the pelvis is inadequate.
- Augmentation is not contraindicated. However, discuss with the consultant before using a Syntocinon (oxytocin) infusion. **Do not use Syntocinon if there is secondary uterine inertia**.
- FBS from the buttock may be performed if fetal distress is suspected – but the only published study suggesting reliability of fetal buttock blood sampling was based on 10 cases only.

44.3.2 Second stage of labour

! Consider CS if there is delay in the second stage.

- If the woman has not had an epidural, then delivery is better conducted in theatre, with the patient prepared for an emergency general anaesthetic.
- Delivery should be conducted by an experienced obstetrician or appropriately trained midwife.
- An anaesthetist and a paediatrician should be present.
- The woman should be placed in the lithotomy position and catheterized.

Allow the breech to descend spontaneously. This is an assisted vaginal delivery, not a breech extraction, so traction should be avoided. Traction could result in extension of the arm and the head, making delivery more difficult.

Unless the perineum is relaxed, perform an episiotomy when the fetal anus is seen over the fourchette. Use a pudendal block if there is no epidural.

The fetal spine usually rotates uppermost. If the legs are extended, then deliver them by flexion at the knee joint and abduction/extension at the hips.

Encourage the mother to push out the breech until the scapulae are visible.

- Cover the baby with a towel.
- Pull down a loop of cord only if necessary.
- Hold the femurs with your thumbs on the sacrum and your other fingers on the anterior superior iliac crest (pelvic-femoral grip), avoiding any pressure on the fetal abdomen.
- Run your finger over the shoulder and down to the elbow to deliver the arm.
- If the arms are extended, gently rotate one shoulder anteriorly and bring the arm down across the chest (Lovset's manoeuvre). The nuchal line should now be visible.

44.3.3 Delivery of the head

- You must see the nape of the neck before proceeding with delivery of the head.
- After an assistant has gently lifted the leg almost to the vertical, deliver with forceps. **Caution**: doing this prematurely could hyperextend the neck and cause damage to the cervical spinal cord.
- Use the Mauriceau–Smellie–Veit manoeuvre if delivery is imminent and there is no time to apply forceps.
- If the head fails to engage, the baby may be allowed to hang for up to 1 minute until the nuchal line is visible (Burns–Marshall technique). Suprapubic pressure can also be applied to guide the head into the pelvis.

44.3.4 Arrest of the after-coming head

This may be due either to entrapment behind an incompletely dilated cervix or to arrest at the pelvic brim. If the cervix is not fully dilated, then incise it at the 4 and/or 8 o'clock positions, taking care not to cut the baby.

For arrest at the pelvic brim, apply suprapubic pressure and/or McRoberts manoeuvre (flexion and abduction of the hips).

44.4 CAESAREAN SECTION FOR BREECH PRESENTATION (ELECTIVE OR EMERGENCY)

Confirm by ultrasound in theatre that the presentation is still breech.

Take care with opening the uterus – scalpel injuries to the baby are more likely to happen in breech than cephalic presentation. A good-size uterine incision is required, particularly in preterm deliveries, to prevent entrapment and traumatic delivery of the baby's head.

External cephalic version

45

External cephalic version (ECV) should be offered to all women with a breech presentation, provided that the following apply:

- Gestational age ≥ 37 weeks.
- There is no contraindication to ECV.
- There is no indication for CS.

45.1 RISKS OF ECV

- Cord accidents
- Fetomaternal transfusion
- Placental abruption
- Rupture of uterus or uterine scar

45.2 CONTRAINDICATIONS TO ECV

- Ruptured membranes
- Vaginal bleeding
- Abnormal CTG
- Rh isoimmunization
- Uterine malformation
- Previous myomectomy
- Placenta praevia
- Multiple pregnancy

45.3 CAUTIONS

ECV may be performed in the following circumstances, but the mother should be informed of the increased risks:

- Previous CS
- Previous episode of bleeding

DOI: 10.1201/9781315099897-51

- IUGR
- Oligohydramnios
- Obesity
- Pre-eclampsia

45.4 ACTION PLAN

- Provide an information leaflet.
- Obtain consent.
- Perform an ultrasound scan to confirm lie and presentation, assess amniotic fluid volume and exclude placenta praevia.
- Perform CTG for 20 minutes before ECV.
- Give a tocolytic: terbutaline 0.25 mg SC about 15 minutes before ECV.
- Version: The breech is lifted out of the pelvis with one hand, and with the other hand pressure is applied to the back of the fetal head to achieve a forward somersault. If this fails, a backward somersault is attempted. Make no more than three attempts at ECV, over 5 minutes.
- After ECV, perform an ultrasound scan to confirm presentation.
- Perform CTG for at least 20 minutes after ECV.
- If the woman is Rh-negative, send a blood sample for a Kleihauer test and give anti-D immunoglobulin 500 units (unless the baby's father is also Rh-negative).
- Proceed to CS if the CTG is abnormal or if the procedure has provoked vaginal bleeding.
- Document CTG observations, tocolytic given, outcome of procedure and further care.
- Agree a follow-up plan:
  - **If ECV is successful**, follow up in the antenatal clinic.
  - **If ECV is unsuccessful**, proceed to elective CS or breech vaginal delivery; document the mother's/couple's decision.

If a woman has had a successful ECV, she should be monitored closely in labour, since there is a higher incidence of CS for various reasons.

The woman with genital cutting

46

While this may occasionally be picked up for the first time in labour, most cases would have been seen and counselled antenatally. Check the notes for any special instructions.

If picked up for the first time:

- Amply document the findings on examination of the vulva (see classification in next section).
- Assess risk: if the unborn child is at risk, report to the designated authority.
- Explain the law.

46.1 WHO CLASSIFICATION OF FEMALE GENITAL CUTTING

Type 1: Partial or total removal of the clitoris and/or the prepuce (clitoridectomy).

Type 2: Partial or total removal of the clitoris and the labia minora, with or without excision of the labia majora (excision).

Type 3: Narrowing of the vaginal orifice with creation of a covering seal by cutting and apposing the labia minora and/or the labia majora, with or without excision of the clitoris (infibulation).

Type 4: All other harmful procedures to the female genitalia for non-medical purposes.

- Anticipate problems and discuss these with the woman:
  - Difficult vaginal examination
  - Difficulty in catheterizing the bladder
  - Difficulty in applying an FSE (if required)
  - Genital tract trauma during delivery
  - Possible need for an anterior midline episiotomy
  - Psychological distress
  - Post-delivery urinary retention (due to pain)
  - Vulvovaginal haematoma

Respect the woman's views and cultural identity and try not to sound patronizing.

46.2 ACTION PLAN

- Offer epidural analgesia: this will facilitate vaginal examination and de-infibulation.
- If vaginal examination is difficult or impossible, the cervix may be assessed by rectal examination, but specific consent for this must be obtained.

DOI: 10.1201/9781315099897-52

- An episiotomy will probably be necessary; this will often be a midline anterior episiotomy in cases of infibulation.
- Provide psychological support postpartum. This may require referral to psychosexual services.
- Check that legal/regulatory requirements have been fulfilled.

> **!** Restoring infibulation (stitching together of the labia) after delivery is illegal under the Female Genital Mutilation Act 2003.

If the baby is female and the family supports female circumcision, social services should be informed. Explain to the woman why this is necessary. Alert the health visitor to possible child-protection issues.

46.3 FEMALE GENITAL MUTILATION ACT 2003

- A person is guilty of an offence if s/he excises, infibulates or otherwise mutilates the whole or any part of a girl's labia majora, labia minora or clitoris.
- A person is guilty of an offence if s/he aids, abets, counsels or procures a girl to excise, infibulate or otherwise mutilate the whole or any part of her own labia majora, labia minora or clitoris.
- The law permits a registered doctor or midwife to perform a surgical operation on a girl who is in any stage of labour, or has just given birth, for purposes connected with the labour or birth. This in practice means the woman can be de-infibulated but not re-infibulated.
- There are similar laws in other countries, for example: Ireland: The Criminal Justice (Female Genital Mutilation) Act 2012 Scotland: Prohibition of Female Genital Mutilation (Scotland) Act 2005 USA: The STOP FGM Act of 2020

The obese woman in labour

47

- Check notes for any plan agreed antenatally.
- Check that the following equipment are available: large blood pressure monitoring cuffs, compression stockings, pneumatic boots, bed, mattress, chair and wheelchair.

$BMI = Weight\ (kg)/(Height\ in\ m)^2$

47.1 WHO CLASSIFICATION OF BMI

Underweight	<18.5
Normal	18.5–24.99
Preobese	25–29.99
Obese Class I	30–34.99
Obese Class II	35–39.99
Obese Class III	>40

The key to reducing intrapartum mortality and morbidity in obese women is anticipatory care in labour. With obese class III women (BMI >40):

- The possibility of missing abnormalities on scans is higher.
- Monitoring the baby in labour is more challenging.
- Siting epidurals could be difficult.
- Surgery is more difficult.
- There is a risk of thromboembolism.
- Breastfeeding is important to help postnatal weight loss.
- Preventative management of pressure sores is important, as there is a higher-than-average chance of a slow labour.
- Ensure adequate hydration.
- A larger operating theatre table is required.
- Alert SpR and anaesthetist on admission.
- Check for any care plan devised antenatally.
- Use an appropriate size sphygmomanometer cuff to measure BP.
- Secure venous access as early as possible. Consider insertion of a second cannula if BMI >40
- Consider insertion of arterial line, especially if pre-eclamptic.
- Group-and-save (increased risk of PPH).
- VTE prophylaxis per protocol. Weight-adjusted dose.
- Anticipate shoulder dystocia.
- Senior obstetrician to be present if CS is required and BMI is >40.

DOI: 10.1201/9781315099897-53

- For prophylactic antibiotic at CS, give a second dose.
- Active management of the third stage (increased risk of PPH).

If there is more than 2 cm subcutaneous fat at CS, the subcutaneous layer should be sutured in order to reduce the risk of wound infection and wound separation.

47.2 WOMAN WHO HAD BARIATRIC SURGERY

- CS is not routinely indicated after bariatric surgery and labour should be managed as outlined previously.
- Pregnancy increases the risk of intestinal obstruction in women who have undergone bariatric surgery, and deaths from it have been reported, so this diagnosis should be excluded if the woman presents with abdominal pain and vomiting.

Perineal tear

48

The perineum should be inspected after every delivery, and the presence or absence of any tear should be documented.

48.1 CLASSIFICATION OF PERINEAL TEARS

- **First degree**: laceration of vaginal epithelium or perineal skin only.
- **Second degree**: also injury to perineal muscles, but not the anal sphincter.
- **Third degree**: disruption of vaginal epithelium, perineal skin, perineal body and anal sphincter muscles:
  - 3a: involving <50% of the thickness of the external sphincter
  - 3b: involving >50% of the thickness of the external sphincter; complete tear of the external sphincter
  - 3c: internal sphincter torn as well
- **Fourth degree**: torn anal sphincter and rectal mucosa.

All tears extending to the anal margin should be regarded as third-degree tears until proven otherwise.

48.2 FIRST- AND SECOND-DEGREE TEARS: EPISIOTOMY

See also Chapter 26.

- Vaginal tears and episiotomies should be repaired with 2/0 Vicryl Rapide.
- Infiltrate with 1% lidocaine, not exceeding 20 mL.
- Care should be taken to start the repair from the apex of the tear.
- For skin closure, a continuous subcuticular suture is associated with less short-term pain than interrupted sutures. Apposing but not suturing the skin is associated with less dyspareunia.

A paravaginal haematoma should be suspected if there are signs of shock after the third stage of labour in the absence of significant bleeding externally. See also Chapter 82.

- A rectal examination should be performed after the repair.
- A swab and needle count should be performed after the repair.
- If there is a substantial periurethral tear, then insert a catheter.

DOI: 10.1201/9781315099897-54

48.3 THIRD- AND FOURTH-DEGREE TEARS

Repair must be performed by an obstetrician trained to do so and must be performed in the operating theatre, with good lighting.

! A general anaesthetic or epidural/spinal is mandatory when there is a third- or fourth-degree tear.

- The anal epithelium should be repaired with Vicryl 3/0 (Ethicon) sutures, either interrupted with the knots tied in the anal lumen or continuous submucosal.
- The internal anal sphincter should be repaired with 3/0 PDS (Ethicon) interrupted sutures.
- The external anal sphincter should be repaired with 3/0 PDS sutures, using either overlapping or end-to-end technique. Bury the surgical knots beneath the superficial perineal muscles to reduce the risk of suture migration to the skin.
- Vaginal repair should be done using Vicryl Rapide.
- Reconstruct the perineal muscles (failure to do so leaves a short, deficient perineum).
- Skin repair should be done using Vicryl Rapide.
- A swab and needle count should be performed after the repair.
- Give cefuroxime 1.5 g and metronidazole 500 mg IV, followed by a 5-day course of oral cefalexin and metronidazole.
- Prescribe:
  - Lactulose 10 mL three times daily for 2 weeks
  - Fybogel, one sachet twice daily for 2 weeks.
- Document the extent of injury and how it was managed. The use of a repair proforma is recommended.
- Arrange a follow-up appointment with a consultant obstetrician and/or perineum clinic, according to the local protocol.

SECTION 2

Medical conditions

Heart disease in labour

49

The Modified World Health Organization (mWHO) classification of maternal cardiovascular risk categorizes various heart conditions as follows:

mWHO class 1: No detectable increased risk of maternal mortality and no or mild increase in morbidity. Example: mild mitral valve prolapse.

mWHO class II: Small increased risk of maternal mortality or moderate increase in morbidity. E.g. unoperated septal defect.

mWHO class II–III: Intermediate increased risk of mortality or moderate to severe increase in morbidity. E.g. Marfan syndrome without aortic dilatation.

WHO class III: Significantly increased risk of maternal mortality or severe morbidity. Expert counselling required. If pregnancy is decided upon, intensive specialist cardiac and obstetric monitoring needed throughout pregnancy, childbirth and the puerperium. E.g. Marfan with aortic dilatation 40–45 mm.

WHO class IV: (pregnancy contraindicated) Extremely high risk of maternal mortality or severe morbidity; pregnancy contraindicated. If pregnancy occurs, termination should be discussed. If pregnancy continues, care as for class III. E.g. Marfan syndrome with aorta dilated >45 mm.

49.1 PRINCIPLES OF MANAGEMENT

Delivery (including place of delivery) must be planned, particularly for women with severe heart disease. Women in mWHO II–III, III and IV risk categories should have their delivery care at a specialized hospital under multidisciplinary supervision.

Liaison between consultant obstetrician, anaesthetist and cardiologist is essential. In most cases, vaginal delivery is preferred to CS. Planned caesarean section is recommended for women with aortic pathology, severe mitral and aortic valve stenosis, intractable heart failure or pulmonary artery hypertension. Urgent caesarean section is indicated for a woman presenting in labour on oral anticoagulants.

The following can be used safely to induce labour:

- Dinoprostone, slow-release formulation of 10 mg (PGE2)
- Dinoprostone 1–3 mg
- Misoprostol 25 µg, prostaglandin E1 (PGE1)

Prevent heart failure – avoid factors that may increase cardiac workload, including:

- Excessive physical effort – use epidural analgesia and prophylactic instrumental delivery
- Anaemia
- Infection
- Hypertension

DOI: 10.1201/9781315099897-56

The following drugs should be avoided: prostaglandin, carboprost, ritodrine, salbutamol
In women with obscure febrile illness, consider the possibility of endocarditis.

49.2 ACTION PLAN

- **Antibiotic cover**: all women in labour and with a structural heart defect, prosthetic valve or a history of endocarditis must have prophylactic antibiotics:
  - **CS**: amoxicillin 1 g IV and gentamicin 120 mg IV (over 3 minutes) at induction of anaesthesia, then amoxicillin 500 mg 6 hours later.
  - **Vaginal delivery**: amoxicillin 1 g IV and gentamicin 120 mg IV (over 3 minutes) at the onset of labour or ruptured membranes, then amoxicillin 500 mg 6 hours later.
  - **If the woman is allergic to penicillin or has had more than a single dose of penicillin in the previous month**: vancomycin 1 g by slow IV infusion (over at least 60 minutes) before delivery, then gentamicin 120 mg IV at induction of anaesthesia or at rupture of membranes.
- Labour should take place in the left lateral or upright position. Avoid supine hypotension.
- ECG (particularly important for women with a history of arrhythmia). Anticipate a need for emergency anti-arrhythmia treatment.
- Pulse oximetry (for early detection of decompensation).
- Administer oxygen by mask, as required.
- Institute continuous CTG.
- Consider arterial line (depending on severity of condition).
- Offer epidural analgesia (avoid systemic hypotension and take care with fluid preloading; avoid if cardiac output is restricted).
- Maintain strictly a fluid balance chart.
- Delay the active phase of the second stage for 2 hours to allow maximal descent of the fetal head, as this will shorten the active phase of the second stage.
- Expedite the second stage of labour (elective forceps or ventouse).
- Third stage of labour: give a slow IV infusion of 2 U of Syntocinon (oxytocin) over 10 min immediately after birth, followed by infusion of 10 units in 500 mL at 36 mL/hr), continued for 4 hours post-delivery.

Do not give ergometrine or Syntometrine (ergometrine with oxytocin).

- If PPH due to atony occurs, misoprostol 600 mcg PR should be used. Avoid high dose Syntocinon and carboprost (Hemabate).
- Ensure thromboembolism prophylaxis, including early ambulation.
- If breastfeeding is contraindicated due to mother's medication, give cabergoline 0.25 mg every 12 h for 2 days.
- Continue high-dependency care for 24–48 hours following delivery: the most dangerous time for the cardiac patient is the first 24 hours after delivery (due to fluid shifts).

Women with Eisenmenger's syndrome need to be in the ITU for at least 7 days after delivery.

49.2.1 Anticoagulant therapy

Some women with cardiac disease will be on anticoagulant therapy – LMWH, unfractionated heparin or oral anticoagulant (warfarin or clopidogrel).

If the woman presents in labour:

- Avoid IM injections.
- Involve the on-call haematologist.
- Stop anticoagulant therapy.
- If she is on UFH and LMWH, give protamine sulphate. Consider repeat dose for the woman on LMWH.

If she is on oral anticoagulant, proceed to CS, to reduce the risk of intracranial bleeding in the baby.

- Give the baby fresh frozen plasma and vitamin K.
- Resume anticoagulants post-delivery if there is no PPH.

49.2.2 Preterm labour

Discuss with the consultant before commencing tocolytics.

Tocolytics, particularly nifedipine, may compromise cardiac function. Atosiban is the preferred tocolytic. Do not use beta-mimetics (salbutamol and ritodrine).

! In patients with heart disease, avoid fluid overload and local anaesthetics containing adrenaline.
! If a pacemaker is in place, do not use unipolar diathermy.

Peripartum cardiomyopathy

50

This is a disease of unknown cause in which left ventricular dysfunction occurs in late pregnancy or puerperium. The condition is rare before 36 weeks. It is characterized by the absence of recognizable heart disease before the last month of pregnancy and the absence of a known cause of heart failure.

50.1 DIAGNOSIS

The aforementioned, plus left ventricular systolic dysfunction on echocardiography.

> ! Any woman without a relevant prior history and who presents with heart failure in late pregnancy should be regarded as having a cardiomyopathy until it is proven otherwise.

50.2 RISK FACTORS

- Advanced age
- Multiparity
- African descent
- Hypertension
- Multiple pregnancy
- Malnutrition
- Smoking
- Diabetes

50.3 SYMPTOMS AND SIGNS

- Breathlessness
- Palpitations
- Swollen legs
- Tachycardia
- Dyspnoea

DOI: 10.1201/9781315099897-57

- Dysrhythmia
- Signs of embolism

This condition could be misdiagnosed as pre-eclampsia.

50.4 ACTION PLAN

- Call for help
- Manage shock: airways, breathing, circulation
- Establish IV access
- FBC, U/E and group-and-save
- Chest X-ray
- ECG
- Echocardiography
- Impose salt and water restriction
- Institute continuous electronic fetal monitoring
- Involve a cardiologist immediately
- Inform a neonatologist
- Inform an anaesthetist
- Institute anticoagulant therapy, diuretics, inotropes and other treatment of heart failure as agreed with the cardiologist

A senior clinician must decide the place, time and mode of delivery. Transfer to a high-risk centre, if feasible. Vaginal delivery is preferable if the woman's condition is stable.

Treatment with bromocriptine (prolactin release inhibitor) may be beneficial.

Pre-eclampsia

51

Pre-eclampsia remains one of the main causes of maternal mortality and morbidity worldwide. It manifests as new hypertension ≥140/90 mmHg and proteinuria ≥2+ on dipstick analysis or >0.3 g/24 h, after 20 weeks' gestation. Women who become hypertensive and either have symptoms or have abnormal haematological or biochemical results should also be regarded as having pre-eclampsia until proven otherwise.

! Not all cases present with the classic features.

Complications of pre-eclampsia include:

- Cerebrovascular accident
- Placental abruption
- HELLP syndrome
- DIC
- Eclampsia
- Hepatic failure
- Renal failure
- Pulmonary oedema
- IUGR

51.1 CLASSIFICATION

Pre-eclampsia is classified as severe if any of the following are seen:
- Dizziness, drowsiness, visual symptoms, epigastric pain/tenderness or chest pain
- Hyperreflexia
- Papilloedema
- Systolic BP >160 mmHg or diastolic BP >110 mmHg
- MAP >125 mmHg
- Proteinuria: 3+ on dipstick or >3 g in a 24-hour urine collection
- Oliguria: <500 mL in 24 hours
- Thrombocytopenia: <100 × 10^9/L
- Creatinine >100 mmol/L
- ALT >50 IU/L
- Pulmonary oedema

DOI: 10.1201/9781315099897-58

'Pre-eclampsia is a disease of signs . . . symptoms are the hallmark of imminent eclampsia.'
Baskett TF. Essential Management of Obstetric Emergencies, 3rd edn.
Bristol: Clinical Press, 1999:79

! Mild pre-eclampsia may progress rapidly to severe disease.
* Fits may occur without any warning signs or symptoms.
* Fits occur more frequently postpartum than intrapartum.

51.2 ACTION PLAN

* Check symptoms
* Check reflexes and fundoscopy
* Obtain hourly BP recording; in women with severe hypertension, record BP every 15–30 minutes until it is less than 160/110 mmHg
* Perform a urinalysis
* FBC
* Group-and-save
* U/E and creatinine
* Urate
* LFT
* Perform a clotting screen
* Insert a 16G Venflon: Hartmann's solution 85 mL/h
* Monitor fluid input and urine output
* Offer epidural analgesia if platelet count >100 × 10⁹/L. Do not preload with intravenous fluids
* Institute continuous electronic fetal monitoring
* Inform consultant obstetrician
* Inform the consultant anaesthetist
* Assess fetal wellbeing: growth, amniotic fluid volume and umbilical artery Doppler ultrasound
* Decide whether to deliver or manage conservatively. This generally entails an evaluation of risks and benefits, but the following is a useful guide:
  * **severe pre-eclampsia**: deliver, regardless of gestational age
  * **mild/moderate pre-eclampsia at term**: deliver
  * **mild/moderate pre-eclampsia preterm**: may be managed conservatively
* If delivery is imminent, give ranitidine 150 mg orally immediately, then 150 mg every 6 hours
* If <34 weeks' gestation, give prophylactic betamethasone for lung maturity
* Commence antihypertensive treatment (see later)

51.3 MEASUREMENT OF BLOOD PRESSURE

Automated BP-monitoring devices are convenient for monitoring trends, but they may underestimate BP. If a device is used, the readings must be checked hourly against sphygmomanometer measurements.

The sphygmomanometer cuff should be at the level of the heart and should be of an appropriate size for the woman. In women whose arm circumference exceeds 35 cm, a large cuff should be used.

Korotkoff sound V (disappearance of the sound) should be used for determining diastolic pressure, not Korotkoff IV (muffling).

51.4 SEVERE PRE-ECLAMPSIA

- Manage in a quiet room and at the appropriate critical care setting. See Table 51.1
- Open a high-dependency care chart
- Connect an ECG monitor
- Connect an O_2 saturation monitor. If O_2 saturation drops below 95%, inform the registrar
- Record BP every 15 minutes; when it is stable, this can be done hourly
- Check the respiratory rate hourly
- Document the EWS
- Insert a Foley catheter and monitor fluid balance
- Commence anticonvulsant prophylaxis (see later)
- Consider insertion of an arterial line. This facilitates precise and continuous monitoring of BP Can be used as an adjunct to non-invasive BP monitoring, particularly in obese women and when there has been a major haemorrhage
- Consider insertion of a CVP line if there is excessive bleeding at delivery and in cases of placental abruption. If CVP <5 cmH$_2$O or >12 cmH$_2$O, then inform the anaesthetist
- If epidural analgesia is accepted, avoid fluid load
- CTG
- If delivery is not imminent, perform an ultrasound scan for fetal growth, amniotic fluid volume and Doppler assessment

! Do not transfer to another hospital unless the woman's clinical condition has been stabilized. Her BP should be below 160/105 mmHg and her oxygen saturation should be normal. (See also in utero transfer, Sections 6.4 to 6.6)

TABLE 51.1   Clinical Criteria for Choice of Critical Care Level

Level 3 care	Severe pre-eclampsia and needing ventilation
Level 2 care	Step-down from level 3 or severe pre-eclampsia with any of the following complications: • eclampsia • HELLP syndrome • haemorrhage • hyperkalaemia • severe oliguria • coagulation support • intravenous antihypertensive treatment • initial stabilization of severe hypertension • evidence of cardiac failure • abnormal neurology
Level 1 care	Pre-eclampsia with hypertension Ongoing conservative antenatal management of severe preterm hypertension Step-down treatment after the birth

51.5 DELIVERY

51.5.1 Timing

Timing of delivery should be judicious. Stabilizing the patient before CS will reduce risks, but delaying delivery could increase risks; each case should be assessed on its merits.

51.5.2 Second stage of labour

If the active phase lasts beyond 30 minutes, advise instrumental delivery.

51.5.3 Third stage of labour

Give Syntocinon (oxytocin) 5 units IV or IM. **Do not use ergometrine or Syntometrine (ergometrine with oxytocin).**

51.6 WATCH FOR PPH

Note that with haemoconcentration, pre-eclamptic patients are less tolerant of haemorrhage than are normotensive women: observe BP and urine output.

51.7 POST-DELIVERY

- Avoid NSAIDs (e.g. diclofenac)
- Manage on the delivery suite until stable
- Maintain vigilance
- Check BP hourly for the first 4 hours, then every 4 hours for 12 hours, and then every 8 hours for 48 hours
- Continue antihypertensive and anticonvulsant treatment as required (see later)
- Give thromboembolism prophylaxis

51.8 ANTIHYPERTENSIVE THERAPY IN PRE-ECLAMPSIA

The aim of treatment is not necessarily to normalize BP but to maintain it at a relatively safe level. If BP drops too low, placental perfusion will be reduced. This is particularly stressful to the growth-restricted fetus. Aim for a MAP <125 mmHg.

- **If systolic BP <160 mmHg, or diastolic BP <105 mmHg, or MAP is in the range 125–140 mmHg**, give oral labetalol 200 mg. Expect BP to drop within 30 minutes.
- **If systolic BP >160 mmHg, or diastolic BP >105 mmHg, or MAP >140 mmHg**, the options are hydralazine or labetalol.

In the author's experience, hydralazine is particularly helpful in women of African descent who are not responsive to labetalol.

51.9 LABETALOL

- Give 200 mg orally, if the woman is able to tolerate oral therapy, or a bolus of 50 mg (10 mL labetalol 5 mg/mL) IV over 10 minutes. This may be repeated at 15-minute intervals up to a maximum of four doses (i.e. 200 mg).
- Follow with a labetalol infusion 5 mg/mL delivered via a syringe pump at a rate of 4 mL/h (20 g/h). Double the rate every 30 minutes until BP is stable and within the target range. The maximum dose is 32 mL/h (160 mg/h).

Side effects of labetalol include headache, postural hypotension (avoid an upright position for 3 hours after IV labetalol) and nausea.

51.9.1 Contraindications to labetalol

- Severe asthma or obstructive airways disease
- Heart block
- Severe peripheral arterial disease

51.10 HYDRALAZINE

- Give hydralazine 5 mg bolus IV over 10 minutes.
- Simultaneously give 500 mL Gelofusine (or other colloid) over 30 minutes.
- If required, follow with a hydralazine infusion 40 mg in 40 mL 0.9% saline, via a syringe pump, starting at 5 mL/h.
- Titrate against BP as follows: double every 30 minutes until stable at a diastolic BP of 90 mmHg or the pulse rate exceeds 130 beats/min; do not exceed 40 mL/h.

Side effects of hydralazine include tachycardia, headache, dizziness, dyspnoea and flushing. These mimic deteriorating pre-eclampsia.

! Do not use hydralazine in women with cardiovascular disease.

When tailing off hydralazine (this is usually post-delivery), halve the infusion rate every 30 minutes.

51.11 NIFEDIPINE

Oral extended-release nifedipine 30 mg daily has been shown to halt progression and reduce intrapartum acute hypertensive therapy among women with severe pre-eclampsia.

51.12 ANTICONVULSANT PROPHYLAXIS IN PRE-ECLAMPSIA

All women with severe pre-eclampsia should receive anticonvulsant prophylaxis.
Loading dose: 4 g

- Take one ampoule of 5 g (mL) magnesium sulphate ($MgSO_4$), and draw 8 mL. Dilute this with 22 mL of 5% dextrose.
- Administer via a syringe pump over 10 minutes (i.e. infusion rate of 180 mL/hour).

Warning: A bolus given too rapidly may cause cardiac arrest

Maintenance dose: 1 g/hour. If she has had a fit, continue for 24 hours after the last fit.

- Take two ampoules of 5 g $MgSO_4$ and dilute in 30 mL of 5% dextrose. This gives a solution of 1 g/5 mL. Infuse via a syringe driven at 5 mL per hour.

Review hourly to ensure that:

- Respiratory rate >12/min
- Urine output >20 mL/h
- Knee or forearm jerk is present
- O_2 saturation ≥95% on air or oxygen

Check serum magnesium level 4 hours after commencing infusion.
If reflexes or respiration is depressed, stop $MgSO_4$ infusion and check the serum magnesium level. See later for management of magnesium toxicity.
If urine output <20 but >10 mL/h, then adjust treatment according to the plasma creatinine level:

- **Normal creatinine (100 mmol/L)**: continue infusion but check the magnesium level every 2 hours.
- **High creatinine (100–150 mmol/L)**: reduce infusion to 0.5 g/h and check the magnesium level every 2 hours.

- **Very high plasma creatinine (>150 mmol/L)**: stop $MgSO_4$ infusion. Check the magnesium level at once and every 2 hours thereafter.

If urine output <10 mL/h, stop $MgSO_4$ infusion.

51.13 MAGNESIUM SULPHATE BLOOD LEVELS

- **Therapeutic**: 2–3.5 mmol/L.
- **Low**: <2 mmol/L. Increase the infusion rate to 2 g/h for 2 hours, then recheck level.
- **High**: 3.5–5.0 mmol/L. Stop infusion. Restart at half the previous rate if urine output >20 mL/h.
- **Very high**: >5.0 mmol/L. Stop infusion. Commence ECG.

51.14 MANAGEMENT OF MAGNESIUM TOXICITY

51.14.1 Features

- Loss of deep tendon reflexes
- Nausea
- Double vision
- Slurred speech
- Respiratory arrest
- Cardiac arrhythmia
- Cardiac arrest (in severe cases)

If magnesium toxicity is suspected:

- Discontinue $MgSO_4$ infusion
- Check magnesium level urgently
- ECG
- If cardiorespiratory arrest is imminent, give 10% calcium gluconate 10 mL IV over 2–5 minutes
- **If cardiac arrest occurs, crash call and cardiopulmonary resuscitation**

51.15 POSTPARTUM

Continue $MgSO_4$ for 24 hours postpartum, or longer if the woman is still hyperreflexic.

- If $MgSO_4$ was commenced post-delivery, continue for 24 hours.
- If she has had a fit, continue $MgSO_4$ for 24 hours after the last fit.

Note: Maternal administration of $MgSO_4$ for longer than 5–7 days in pregnancy has been associated with skeletal adverse effects and hypocalcaemia and hypermagnesemia in neonates.

Continue antihypertensives until diastolic BP <100 mmHg or MAP <125 mmHg.

51.16 POST-DELIVERY WARD ROUND (DAYS 0–3)

It is important for doctors and midwives to remain alert after delivery, since some women may suffer a postnatal deterioration. A fit may occur for the first time postnatally.

- Check temperature, pulse, BP and respiratory rate. Chart EWS
- Check O_2 saturation. If O_2 saturation <95% or respiratory rate >25/min, request a chest X-ray
- Assess sensorium. Abnormal sensorium with hyperreflexia is indicative of cerebral oedema
- Check fluid balance
- Exclude abnormal bleeding
- FBC and coagulation screen every 8 hours for the first 24 hours
- LFT daily
- Suspect hepatic rupture if right upper quadrant pain is persistent: arrange a CT scan
- Medication: do current doses of antihypertensive and other medication need to be adjusted

51.17 FLUID MANAGEMENT IN PRE-ECLAMPSIA

51.17.1 Principles

Problems related to excessive fluids (pulmonary oedema and ARDS) are much more common than those related to inadequate fluids. ARDS is a frequent mode of death from hypertensive disorders of pregnancy.

In severe pre-eclampsia, there is an increase in systemic vascular resistance. Vasodilator therapy can reduce this, resulting in precipitate hypotension and poor end-organ perfusion. Vasodilator therapy should therefore be accompanied by a fluid load to maintain or improve organ (placenta and kidneys) perfusion.

In severe pre-eclampsia, BP may be maintained despite regional blockade. Do not preload with fluids before epidural in anticipation of hypotension.

Oedema mobilizes back into the circulation within 24–36 hours after delivery.

Patients with excessive haemorrhage require totally different management, including invasive monitoring in many cases.

51.17.2 Pre-delivery

- Background fluids: Hartmann's solution 85 mL/h.
- If Syntocinon infusion has been given, the volume should be included in the calculation of fluid input. *Note*: if a woman with severe pre-eclampsia requires a Syntocinon infusion, a high concentration (30 units in 500 mL 0.9% saline) should be used (Table 51.2).

TABLE 51.2 Syntocinon Infusion Regimen for Women With Severe Pre-Eclampsia

TIME AFTER STARTING (MIN)	AMOUNT OF SYNTOCINON INFUSED (MILLIUNITS/MIN)	VOLUME INFUSED (ML/H)
0	2	2
30	4	4
60	8	8
90	12	12
120	16	16
150	20	20
180	24	24
210	28	28
240	32	32

- Correct any pre-existing fluid deficits (due e.g. to a long period of nil by mouth, vomiting or blood loss).
- Maintain a strict fluid input/urine output chart.
- Give a fluid bolus of 500 mL Gelofusine or Haemaccel over 30 minutes before or at the same time as:
  - Loading with magnesium sulphate.
  - Loading with intravenous hydralazine or if urine output <100 mL in 4 hours.

! Diuretics (e.g. furosemide 10–20 mg) are not appropriate except in pulmonary oedema.

! Do not give any woman more than two fluid boluses, unless she is bleeding.

Delivery is indicated if there is:

- Pulmonary oedema
- Renal failure (rising urea/creatinine)
- Irreversible oliguria despite the aforementioned measures.

51.17.3 Post-delivery

- Ensure that peripartum losses have been replaced. Note that a natural diuresis occurs postpartum.
- Background fluids: Hartmann's solution 50 mL/h for 24 hours, then 80 mL/h. Total fluid input in the first 24 hours should not exceed 2 L.
- Replace any continuing loss. Check U/E (watch for hyponatraemia).
- Look for signs of pulmonary oedema: rising respiratory rate and heart rate, O_2 saturation <95% on air, chest signs and abnormal chest X-ray. If present, give furosemide as note earlier, whatever the urine output. Also give oxygen.

- CVP monitoring will usually be required in patients with significant haemorrhage, renal failure or pulmonary oedema that does not respond rapidly to normal therapeutic measures.

51.18 MANAGEMENT OF OLIGURIA (<80 ML IN 4 HOURS)

- **If the woman is hypovolaemic (see next section) or bleeding**, replace loss.
- **If the woman is not hypovolaemic (see next section) and not bleeding**:
  - Provided that there are no signs of fluid overload and that fluid input in the last 24 hours has not exceeded output by >750 mL, give 200 mL IV fluid (colloid) over 30 minutes. If urine output does not improve, give furosemide 10 mg IV.
  - If fluid input exceeds output by >750 mL, do not give colloid infusion; give furosemide 10 mg IV.
  - If oliguria persists, consult a renal physician.

51.18.1 Features of hypovolaemia

- Dry mouth
- Loss of skin turgor
- Cold extremities
- Raised pulse rate
- Hypotension
- Reduced pulse pressure
- Raised respiratory rate

! Tachypnoea could also be a sign of fluid overload (pulmonary oedema).

51.19 BLOOD TRANSFUSION

Blood transfusion may increase the intravascular oncotic pressure and cause pulmonary oedema in a woman with severe pre-eclampsia. Unless it is absolutely necessary (e.g. acute blood loss), transfusion should be withheld until after diuresis has occurred.

Eclampsia

52

Management aims to:

- Control convulsions
- Control BP
- Deliver the baby

Beware of postpartum eclampsia (see later).

52.1 ACTION PLAN

- Maintain the airway
- Turn the patient to the left lateral position
- Administer oxygen by mask (at least 10 L/min)
- Insert an IV line
- Arrest convulsions with $MgSO_4$. Diazepam 10 mg IV may also be used
- Prevent further fits with $MgSO_4$ infusion
- Treat hypertension

52.2 ANTICONVULSANT TREATMENT (MAGNESIUM SULPHATE)

52.2.1 Loading dose: 4 g

- Take one ampoule of 5 g (mL) magnesium sulphate ($MgSO_4$) and draw 8 mL. Dilute this with 22 mL of 5% dextrose.
- Administer via a syringe pump over 10 minutes (i.e. infusion rate of 180 mL/hour).

Warning: a bolus given too rapidly may cause cardiac arrest.

52.2.2 Maintenance dose: 1 g/hour

- Take two ampoules of 5 g $MgSO_4$ and dilute in 30 mL of 5% dextrose. This gives a solution of 1 g/5 mL. Infuse via a syringe driven at 5 mL per hour.

DOI: 10.1201/9781315099897-59

If venous access not achieved, consider IM administration of magnesium sulphate: loading dose of 10 g (5 g IM in each buttock), followed by 5 g every 4 hours. IM magnesium sulphate is painful, so mix this with 1 mL of xylocaine 2% solution.

Note that the rate of adverse effects is higher with IM administration.

Review hourly to ensure that:

- Respiratory rate >12/min
- Urine output >20 mL/h
- Knee or forearm jerk is present
- O_2 saturation ≥95%

! If convulsions recur, give 2 g (10 mL) 20% $MgSO_4$ solution over 5 minutes.

The maintenance dose should be continued for 24 hours after the last seizure.

Side effects of $MgSO_4$ infusion include double vision, slurred speech, respiratory depression, loss of tendon reflexes, cardiac arrhythmia and cardiac arrest.

If reflexes or respiration are depressed, stop $MgSO_4$ infusion and check serum magnesium level. Respiratory depression should be treated with calcium gluconate 1 g (**10 mL** of **10%** calcium gluconate) IV given over **10 minutes**.

If urine output <20 but >10 mL/h, adjust treatment according to the plasma creatinine level:

- **Normal creatinine (100 mmol/L)**: continue infusion but check the magnesium level every 2 hours.
- **High creatinine (100–150 mmol/L)**: reduce infusion to 0.5 g/h and check the magnesium level every 2 hours.
- **Very high plasma creatinine (>150 mmol/L)**: stop $MgSO_4$ infusion. Check magnesium level at once and every 2 hours thereafter.

If urine output <10 mL/h, stop $MgSO_4$ infusion ($MgSO_4$ is mostly excreted in urine, so oliguria could be associated with toxicity).

52.3 MAGNESIUM SULPHATE BLOOD LEVELS

- **Therapeutic**: 2–3.5 mmol/L.
- **Low**: <2 mmol/L. Increase the infusion rate to 2 g/h for 2 hours, then recheck level.
- **High**: 3.5–5 mmol/L. Stop infusion. Restart at half the previous rate if urine output >20 mL/h.
- **Very high**: >5 mmol/L. Stop infusion. Commence ECG.

52.4 PERSISTENT SEIZURES

If seizures persist despite magnesium:

- Try diazepam 10 mg IV.
- An anaesthetist may give thiopentone 50 mg IV.

- Consider intubating the patient.
- Further seizures should be managed by intermittent positive-pressure ventilation and muscle relaxation.
- If the fits are refractory, a CT or MRI scan should be performed.

52.5 CONTROLLING BLOOD PRESSURE

This is as for management of hypertension in pre-eclampsia.

- Avoid a precipitous drop in BP.

52.6 GENERAL MANAGEMENT

This is as for pre-eclampsia (Chapter 51).

- A decision must be made immediately regarding mode of delivery.
- After delivery, the woman should remain in high dependency care until at least 24 hours have elapsed without a fit.
- Anticonvulsant therapy should be continued until 24 hours have elapsed since the last fit and the woman is no longer hyperreflexic.
- Fluid management is as for pre-eclampsia (see Sections 51.17 and 51.18).

! If there are focal neurological signs, then CT or MRI scan of the brain should be performed.

! One woman had a seizure in hospital after a CS for pre-eclampsia at term and appeared to be making a good recovery but was found collapsed and pulseless after being left unattended in a bath on the fourth day after delivery.
Why Mothers Die. *Report on Confidential Enquiries into Maternal Deaths in the UK, 1994–96.* London: The Stationery Office, 1998:39

Diabetes mellitus

53

53.1 RECOMMENDED TIMING OF DELIVERY

- Type 1 or type 2 diabetes and no other complications: elective birth by induced labour or (if indicated) caesarean section, between 37 weeks and 38 weeks plus 6 days of pregnancy.
- Type 1 or type 2 diabetes with metabolic or other maternal or fetal complications: elective birth before 37 weeks.
- Gestational diabetes without complications: elective birth by induced labour or (if indicated) by caesarean section to women who have not given birth by 40 weeks + 6 days.
- Gestational diabetes with maternal or fetal complications: elective birth before 40 weeks + 6 days.

Details of intrapartum management will usually have been decided in the joint diabetic clinic and written in the case notes.

Management will depend on the presence or absence of complications and whether the woman is on insulin. Women with type 1 or type 2 diabetes and no other complications are advised to have an elective birth by induced labour or (if indicated) caesarean section, between 37 weeks and 38 weeks plus 6 days of pregnancy.

Induction of labour or CS in a diabetic woman should be performed first thing in the morning.

53.2 INDUCTION OF LABOUR BY ARTIFICIAL RUPTURE OF FETAL MEMBRANES

- The woman should have her usual dose of insulin the evening before.
- She should be nil by mouth from midnight.
- At 0800, perform ARM and commence insulin/glucose protocol (see later).

53.3 INDUCTION OF LABOUR WITH PROSTAGLANDIN

- Allow the patient to eat and drink.
- The woman should have her usual dose of insulin until she is in established labour.
- Commence insulin/glucose protocol when she is in established labour.

DOI: 10.1201/9781315099897-60

53.4 ELECTIVE CAESAREAN SECTION

- The woman should have a bedtime snack the night before, then nil by mouth.
- She should have her usual evening dose of insulin, or as prescribed by the diabetologist.
- The morning dose of insulin should be skipped.
- CS should be performed in the morning (first on the list).
- A sliding scale of insulin should be given in theatre (women with gestational diabetes are unlikely to need this).
- If she has general anaesthesia, monitor blood glucose every 30 minutes from induction of general anaesthesia until after the baby is born and she is fully conscious.

53.5 FIRST STAGE OF LABOUR

- Institute continuous fetal monitoring.
- Recommend epidural analgesia.
- FBC, U/E, group-and-save.
- Check urine for ketones.
- Insert two IV lines:
    - **Line 1**: 5% glucose + 10 mmol KCl 500 mL at 100 mL/h through an infusion pump (for a pre-eclamptic patient on fluid restriction, use 10% glucose at 40 mL/h).
    - **Line 2**: 0.9% saline 50 mL + short-acting insulin 50 units (i.e. a concentration of 1 unit/mL), via a pump according to a sliding scale (Table 53.1) (for a pre-eclamptic patient on fluid restriction, use 25 units in 50 mL).
    Note: If the woman opts to use her insulin pump (continuous subcutaneous insulin infusion (CSII)) in labour, IV access should still be obtained (in anticipation of possible IV insulin therapy or treatment of severe hypoglycaemia).
- Check capillary blood glucose hourly. The meter used for capillary blood glucose measurement should be checked by comparing a capillary reading with the value obtained for a venous sample sent to the laboratory – the readings should not differ by more than 1.0 mmol/L.

TABLE 53.1   Sliding Scale for Insulin Infusion

BLOOD GLUCOSE CONCENTRATION (MMOL/L)	INSULIN INFUSION RATE (UNITS/H)
≤2	0
2.1–3.9	0.5
4.0–6.9	1
7.0–8.9	2
9.0–10.9	4
11.0–16	6
>16	8

Aim to keep the blood glucose concentration in the range 4–7 mmol/L.

- If blood glucose is below this range, give glucose (e.g. 60 mL Lucozade, 100 mL Ribena or IV 10% glucose 150 mL) and recheck blood glucose.
- If blood glucose falls outside this range 3 hours after starting the sliding scale, call the diabetologist.

There should be a dedicated IV line for insulin – no other medication should be given through this line.

- Use separate IV access for IV Syntocinon (oxytocin) or preloading for epidural.
- Before commencing insulin infusion, prime the tubing with about 20 mL of the insulin solution.
- The infusion pump and lines should be checked every hour.

⚠ **Be cautious with the use of a three-way tap for glucose/insulin infusions because inadvertent disconnection of one line could be disastrous.**

! Always check that the glucose drip is working.

If there are difficulties with blood glucose control, check the following:

- The pump may not be working.
- The glucose drip may not be working or may be running into tissue.
- Syntocinon may have been added to glucose instead of to saline.

! If Syntocinon is required, it should be via saline infusion, not glucose.

Beware of secondary arrest, in view of possible macrosomia.
If shoulder dystocia is anticipated:

- Discuss this with the woman.
- Revise the shoulder dystocia drill now.

53.6 GESTATIONAL DIABETES, DIET-CONTROLLED

- Check blood glucose on admission and then hourly:
  - **If blood glucose <3.9 mmol/L or labour lasts >8 hours**, commence dextrose 5% infusion.
  - **If blood glucose >7 mmol/L**, commence insulin/glucose protocol (see earlier). Insulin may be needed in the second stage of labour owing to a catecholamine surge.
- On the day after delivery, check blood glucose levels: preprandial, 2 hours after lunch and at bedtime.
- Arrange a glucose tolerance test at 6–8 weeks post-delivery.

53.7 PRETERM LABOUR

See also Chapters 37 and 38.

- Manage according to the diabetic protocol.
- Ritodrine should not be used.
- Betamethasone may affect blood glucose control – so avoid if glucose control on admission is poor. If glucose control on admission is satisfactory, the effect of dexamethasone can be controlled by increasing the dose of SC insulin in consultation with the diabetologist.

53.8 AFTER DELIVERY

Perform capillary blood glucose monitoring every 2 hours.

53.8.1 Gestational diabetes

- Discontinue insulin/glucose infusion once the woman is able to eat a light diet.
- Discontinue any glucose-lowering medication.
- She may eat and drink a normal diet without SC insulin.

53.8.2 Type 1 and type 2 diabetes

- Once the placenta is delivered, reduce the insulin dose by 50%.
- Continue the sliding-scale infusion until the woman is able to eat and drink.
- The first SC dose of insulin should overlap the IV infusion by 30 minutes.
- Monitor blood glucose pre-meal and at bedtime.
- Restart SC insulin on the pre-pregnancy dose. If this is not known, seek advice from the diabetologist.
- If the woman was on oral hypoglycaemic agents prior to her pregnancy, check whether this is compatible with breastfeeding.
- If she was on insulin, explain that there is an increased risk of hypoglycaemia in the postnatal period, especially when breastfeeding. She should have a meal/snack before feeds.

Do not transfer to the postnatal ward until blood glucose levels are normal and there is no ketonuria.

53.9 CARE OF THE NEONATE

- Routine blood glucose test 2–4 hours after birth.
- Feed the baby within 30 minutes of birth and then every 2–3 hours, to maintain a pre-feed capillary plasma glucose level of at least 2.0 mmol/litre.
- The baby should be transferred to the neonatal unit if any of the following is observed:

- Hypoglycaemia associated with clinical signs
- Respiratory distress
- Signs of cardiac or neurological abnormality

53.10 MATERNAL HYPOGLYCAEMIC SHOCK

! **Call for help**: anaesthetist and endocrinologist on call.

Do a quick dipstick test to determine whether this is hypoglycaemia (<2.5 mmol/L) or ketoacidosis (usually, but not always, >9 mmol/L).

Manage shock: airways, breathing, circulation.

☐ Institute continuous electronic fetal monitoring.
☐ Give 50 mL of 50% glucose IV.
☐ Chart vital signs and O_2 saturation.
☐ Repeat finger-prick glucose every 30 minutes.

53.11 DIABETIC KETOACIDOSIS

Risk factors include infection, stress and the use of steroids to accelerate fetal lung maturity.

53.12 PRESENTATION

- Nausea
- Vomiting
- Polydipsia
- Dizziness
- Air hunger
- Tachycardia
- Tachypnoea
- Hypotension
- Smell of ketones

! **Call for help**: anaesthetist and endocrinologist on call.

The woman needs high-dependency or intensive care. The consultant anaesthetist and diabetologist should be engaged in the management of this condition.

Do a quick dipstick glucose test to confirm that this is ketoacidosis (usually, but not always, >9 mmol/L), rather than hypoglycaemia (<2.5 mmol/L).

Manage shock: airways, breathing, circulation.

- Institute continuous electronic fetal monitoring
- Chart vital signs and O_2 saturation
- Blood tests: FBC, glucose, U/E, group-and-save, blood culture and arterial blood gases
- Obtain a midstream specimen of urine for bacteriology
- Urinalysis
- Insert a Foley catheter: monitor fluid input and urine output
- Insert a nasogastric tube (to reduce the risk of aspiration)
- Treat dehydration: IV infusion of 0.9% saline
- Check capillary blood glucose hourly
- Administer insulin as advised by the physician (usually a loading dose of 10 units insulin, followed by an infusion of 5–10 units/h)
- Give 20–40 mmol of potassium in each litre of 0.9% saline, over 3 hours
- Treat infection, if present
- If the woman is undelivered, determine the time and mode of delivery
- Alert the paediatricians

Asthma (acute exacerbation in labour)

54

Women with well-controlled asthma usually have healthy pregnancies, normal labour and good perinatal outcomes and should be advised to continue their usual asthma medication in labour. Acute exacerbation of asthma in labour is rare but should be treated aggressively when it occurs. It can be precipitated by stress, medication (see next) or upper respiratory tract infection.

54.1 DRUGS THAT CAN CAUSE OR AGGRAVATE BRONCHOSPASM

- Ergometrine
- NSAIDs (e.g. diclofenac)
- Aspirin sensitivity
- Beta-blockers (e.g. labetalol)
- Prostaglandin F_2 analogues (carboprost/Hemabate)

Note: prostaglandin E_2 and oxytocin are safe.

54.2 ACTION POINTS

- Document pulse rate, respiratory rate and EWS: respiratory rate >25/min and pulse rate >110 beats/min are consistent with exacerbation
- Record oxygen saturation
- Check peak expiratory flow (PEF). This is a measure of how fast the patient can breathe out (exhale) air: it is the amount of air that she can forcibly blow out in 1 second, measured in litres. PEF <50% of predicted normal is consistent with severe exacerbation. PEF <33% of predicted normal is indicative of life-threatening exacerbation
- Chest X-ray
- FBC
- U/E
- Arterial blood gas analysis:
  - Hypercapnia: $PaCO_2$ >kPa
  - Hypoxia: PaO_2 <8 kPa
  - Acidosis

DOI: 10.1201/9781315099897-61

If any of the aforementioned occur, then repeat the test 30–60 minutes after commencement of treatment.

- Administer oxygen to achieve an O_2 saturation ≥95%
- CTG
- Exclude differential diagnoses: pulmonary embolism (PE), pulmonary oedema, cardiac disease and aspiration
- Avoid morphine; use fentanyl instead
- Recommend epidural as it decreases oxygen consumption and reduces hyperventilation
- Consult a medical specialist
- Administer a bronchodilator: beta-agonist, e.g. salbutamol via nebulizer
- Administer corticosteroid: inhaled, oral or IV. Prednisolone 30–50 mg orally, or hydrocortisone 100 mg IV

If there is no response to treatment, then admission to the ICU is indicated.

Women who have used oral steroids for >2 weeks prior to delivery should be given hydrocortisone 100 mg IV every 6–8 hours to cover the stress of the labour. The reason for this is that theoretically the prolonged use of systemic steroids could suppress the hypothalamic–pituitary axis, with the result that the usual release of adrenal corticosteroids during labour does not occur and symptoms of adrenal insufficiency may be observed during or after delivery.

54.3 AFTER DELIVERY

- Breastfeeding is not contraindicated.
- Physiotherapy should be given.
- Administer salbutamol 2.5–5 mg via a nebulizer.
- In severe cases, consider an IV bronchodilator:
    - Aminophylline 250 mg/30 min
    - Salbutamol 200 µg/10 min
    - Terbutaline 200 µg/10 min

Epilepsy

55

55.1 MANAGEMENT IN LABOUR

- Reassure that most women with epilepsy will have a normal, vaginal delivery.
- Continue the usual anticonvulsant regimen during labour and postpartum. If vomiting occurs within 1 hour of ingestion, administer the same dose again.
- Discuss pain control. Pethidine is contraindicated since it is metabolized to norpethidine, which could trigger a fit. Instead, use diamorphine.
- Inadequate analgesia induces hyperventilation (which could trigger a fit).
- Avoid sleep deprivation, exhaustion and dehydration – these may trigger fits. Fits may also be triggered by bright flickering lights, noise, lack of sleep and emotional stress.
- The woman must not be left on her own.
- If the woman has had a previous seizure in labour or is at increased risk of seizures (e.g. owing to stress or fear), she can be given oral clobazam 10 mg (a long-acting benzodiazepine), two doses 12 hours apart.
- Give appropriate support in cases of congenital malformation or dysmorphic features.
- Check that resuscitation equipment is readily available.

55.2 INDICATIONS FOR CAESAREAN SECTION

- Status epilepticus
- Uncontrolled repeated seizures
- Fetal distress

55.3 MANAGEMENT OF FITS IN LABOUR

- **Call for help.**
- Place the woman in a wedged position (to avoid vena cava compression).
- Keep her head lower than her body, to allow any vomit to drain.
- Clear her airways.
- Administer oxygen by facemask.
- Give IV lorazepam 4 mg bolus. If required, a further 1 mg bolus is given slowly. Use a large vein.

- Alternatively, give IV diazepam 10 mg; further 2 mg boluses may be given if required, but do not exceed a total of 20 mg. However, lorazepam is less sedative, and so associated with a lower risk of aspiration.
- If this fails to control seizures (i.e. the woman is in status epilepticus), give IV phenytoin 15 mg/kg at an infusion rate $\leq$ 50 mg/min.
- In status epilepticus, endotracheal intubation may be required.

- **Do not** leave the woman unattended.
- **Do not** restrain her.
- **Do not** put anything in her mouth.
- **Do not** give her anything by mouth until you are certain that she is fully recovered.

55.4 AFTER SEIZURE

- Reassure the woman when she recovers
- Make her comfortable (she may have had involuntary loss of urine during seizure)
- CTG

If there is doubt whether a seizure in labour is due to eclampsia or epilepsy, then, in addition to IV lorazepam or diazepam, a slow IV bolus of 4 g magnesium sulphate over 5–10 minutes followed by 1 g/h for 24 hours is recommended.

55.5 AFTER DELIVERY

The mother needs sleep. Postnatal exhaustion and sleep deprivation may precipitate seizures. A short course of oral clobazam 10 mg nocte for 2–4 days can be given if necessary.

- Vitamin K 1 mg should be given to the baby at birth if the mother has been using enzyme-inducing anticonvulsant medication.

Encourage breastfeeding but support the woman in her choice of feeding method. Anticonvulsant drugs are excreted in breast milk in low concentrations, but the risks to the baby (irritability and lethargy) are minor compared with the benefits of breastfeeding. However, if the mother is on lamotrigine, warn her that the baby may have a skin rash, in which case breastfeeding will have to be discontinued.

! Fits can occur in the immediate postnatal period, resulting in accidents to mother and baby.

- Give advice regarding infant care to minimize danger to the baby in the event of the mother having a fit. Accidents can also occur during a bath or shower, so a midwife or health worker should be aware and the door should not be locked.
- Review anticonvulsant medication and discuss contraception.

With the woman's consent, report to the UK Epilepsy and Pregnancy Register, Dept. of Neurology, Level 6 OPC, Royal Victoria Hospital, Grosvenor Rd. Belfast BT12 6BA. Tel (free-of-charge): 0800 389 1248. www.epilepsyandpregnancy.co.uk

Systemic lupus erythematosus

56

56.1 PRINCIPLES

Systemic lupus erythematosus (SLE) is an immunological disorder in which antibodies are formed against the body's own DNA and other cellular components. It is characterized by vasculitis and antinuclear antibodies. Other manifestations include cutaneous and neurological signs. The woman may present on the delivery suite with fetal growth restriction, intrauterine fetal demise, pre-eclampsia, IUGR or preterm labour.

The following are associated with increased risk of adverse outcome in pregnancy: active disease; hypertension; kidney dysfunction; antiphospholipid antibodies; anti-Ro or anti-La antibodies.

- Implement a plan agreed and documented antenatally.
- Watch for:
    - Acute exacerbation in labour
    - Hypertension
    - Thrombosis
    - Congenital heart block
    - Neonatal lupus
- Features of a flare include fever, arthralgia, myalgia, rash, oral ulcers and hypertension.

It may be difficult to distinguish lupus flare from pre-eclampsia. Features common to both conditions include hypertension, proteinuria, oedema, thrombocytopenia and renal dysfunction.

Note that pre-eclampsia may coexist with lupus flare. In lupus flare, urine microscopy shows red blood cells, leukocytes and granular casts.

- Transfer of antibodies across the placenta may result in congenital heart block.
- A paediatrician should be present at delivery.
- CS should be performed for obstetric indications.

56.2 ACTION PLAN

- Institute continuous electronic fetal monitoring
- Check FBC, serum urate, creatinine, urea and electrolytes on admission
- Urinalysis
- Monitor hourly urine output
- Alert an anaesthetist

DOI: 10.1201/9781315099897-63

- Alert a paediatrician
- Liaise with a rheumatologist and the immunology laboratory
- If the woman is on long-term steroid therapy, give hydrocortisone 100 mg IV every 8 hours (three doses) because of inhibition of the pituitary–adrenal axis
- If acute exacerbation occurs, discuss management with the medical team. Steroids may be required

After delivery, consider doubling her usual dose of prednisolone for 2–3 days.

- Hydroxychloroquine, azathioprine and steroids are safe for breastfeeding.
- In respect of discontinuation and resumption of anticoagulant therapy.

56.3 NEONATAL LUPUS

This syndrome comprises congenital heart block, transient cutaneous lupus lesions and systemic manifestations. It is caused by antibodies (anti-SSA/Ro and/or anti-SSB/La) passed across the placenta from mother to baby, but only about 1% of women who have these autoantibodies will have a baby with neonatal lupus.

- It occurs in 5% of babies born to women with SLE.
- Neonatal lupus also occurs in babies of women who do not have SLE.

Connective tissue disorders

57

! If the woman is on long-term steroid therapy, give hydrocortisone 100 mg IV every 8 hours (three doses) because of inhibition of the pituitary–adrenal axis.

57.1 RHEUMATOID ARTHRITIS

- If the woman has been on NSAIDs, watch for peripartum haemorrhage. NSAIDs should be avoided after week 32 due to a risk of closure of fetal ductus arteriosus in utero.
- Watch for pre-eclampsia.
- If woman is unable to fully abduct the hip, this may impede vaginal delivery.
- In the absence of pelvic joint deformity, aim for vaginal birth.
- Rarely, atlanto-axial subluxation complicates general anaesthesia.
- Institute continuous electronic fetal monitoring.
- Breastfeeding is not contraindicated. Due to pain, mother may need help in positioning the baby comfortably for breastfeeding.

57.2 MARFAN SYNDROME

The main risk is that of aortic dissection in labour. Watch out for symptoms of possible dissection: chest/abdominal/upper back pain; weakness; difficulty in breathing or speaking; loss of consciousness.

- Institute continuous electronic fetal monitoring.
- Check the notes for a plan agreed with the cardiologist.
- Have an anaesthetic plan in advance.
- If aortic root diameter >4 cm, then recommend elective CS (because there is a 10% risk of aortic dissection in labour/delivery).
- Vaginal delivery is possible in uncomplicated cases. Forceps delivery to shorten the second stage of labour is recommended.
- If the woman has heart-valve incompetence, give prophylactic antibiotics (Chapter 75).

DOI: 10.1201/9781315099897-64

57.3 EHLERS–DANLOS SYNDROME

This is a group of 13 inherited disorders of collagen metabolism, characterized by fragile skin and blood vessels and by hypermobility of the joints. Management in labour is individualized, as appropriate to the type and severity of the condition.

Women with types I (classical) and IV (vascular) disease are more likely to develop complications in pregnancy, with a mortality rate of 20%–25% in type IV disease. PROM occurs frequently.

Malpresentation in labour is common, and the baby may be growth-restricted.

Potential problems include rupture of the great vessels during labour, vaginal and perineal tears, rupture of the scar in women with previous CS, difficulties with intubation, uterine rupture, PPH, delayed wound healing and genital prolapse.

The mode of delivery should be decided by the consultant in discussion with the woman.

Support group: Hypermobility Syndromes Association. 49 Greek Street, London, W1D 4EG. Helpline +44 (0)33 3011 6388 info@hypermobility.org

SECTION 3

Haemorrhage and haematological disorders

The rhesus-negative woman

58

Approximately 60% of babies born to Rh(D)-negative women in the UK are Rh-positive. Sensitized Rh-negative women with a significant antibody titre will usually be transferred to a tertiary centre. **The following applies to *non-sensitized* women.**

58.1 SENSITIZING EVENTS

Following any potentially sensitizing event, such as trauma, placental abruption, vaginal bleeding, external cephalic version (ECV) or amniocentesis:

* Give anti-D immunoglobulin 500–1000 units.
* Carry out a Kleihauer test, and then give additional anti-D if indicated.

58.2 AT DELIVERY

* The midwife who conducts delivery or receives the baby in theatre should obtain cord and maternal blood within 2 hours of delivery for (a) ABO and Rh(D) typing and (b) screening test for fetal maternal haemorrhage.
* If unable to obtain cord blood, the midwife must perform a heel prick before the mother and baby are transferred to the postnatal ward.

All previously non-sensitized Rh-negative women who have given birth to a Rh-positive baby should be given 500–1000 IU anti-D within 72 hours of delivery.

Following intrauterine fetal death (where a sample was not obtained from the baby), administer 500–1000 IU anti-D Ig to D negative, previously non-sensitized women within 72 h of the diagnosis of IUFD.

Following use of intraoperative cell salvage (ICS) at caesarean delivery (baby confirmed to be Rh(D)-positive or status unknown):

* Administer 1500 IU anti-D Ig after the reinfusion of salvaged red cells.
* Test for FMH 30–45 min after reinfusion in case more anti-D Ig is indicated.
* Liaise with the transfusion laboratory so that the correct dose of anti-D Ig is issued.

DOI: 10.1201/9781315099897-66

58.3 TRANSFUSIONS

Rh(D)-negative women of childbearing potential should receive Rh(D)-negative platelets. If unavailable, Rh(D)-positive platelets can be given with anti-D prophylaxis. If an Rh(D)-negative woman receives a platelet transfusion, check the product to confirm whether it is Rh-positive or Rh-negative platelets. If it is Rh(D)-positive, then anti-D should be given (discuss dose with the haematologist).

If an Rh(D)-negative woman receives Rh(D)-positive blood in error, discontinue the transfusion immediately. Send a maternal blood specimen for estimation of the volume of Rh(D)-positive cells in circulation. Give anti-D 500 units for every 4 mL of Rh(D)-positive blood transfused. Refer to the local protocol for managing transfusion errors.

CLINICAL SAFETY INCIDENT FROM THE 2021 ANNUAL SHOT REPORT:

PATIENT DISCHARGED BEFORE BEING GIVEN ANTI-D IMMUNOGLOBULIN (IG)

The patient had a vaginal bleed at 38+6 weeks gestation and attended maternity triage the same evening. A sample was taken for a Kleihauer test and a standard dose of anti-D Ig was issued by the laboratory.

As Kleihauer tests are not routinely completed overnight at this hospital, the standard dose should have been given with a follow-up once Kleihauer result is available, if more anti-D Ig is required. However, the patient was sent home without the standard dose being given because the doctor was waiting for the Kleihauer result before giving any anti-D Ig.

The midwife was asked to write the patient's details in the follow-up diary to be contacted the next day, which she did. Unfortunately, the midwife on duty the following day overlooked this in the diary. The patient was therefore not contacted. The anti-D Ig was found in the blood refrigerator during subsequent checks. The patient had not been given a date or time to attend for anti-D Ig administration by the discharging doctor, neither had she been contacted by the midwives. The anti-D Ig was administered but beyond the required 72-hour period.

Thromboembolism prophylaxis

59

All women, irrespective of history, should have general measures (mobilization and avoidance of dehydration) to minimize the risk of VTE.

Specific thromboprophylaxis is indicated in:

- All patients undergoing CS.
- Women in normal labour and with a history of thrombosis, thrombophilia or other risk factors.

If the woman had received antenatal prophylaxis, no further low molecular weight heparin (LMWH) should be injected once labour commences.

Where dalteparin 5000 IU is specified in this book for thromboprophylaxis, the following alternative LMWH could be used:

- Enoxaparin, 40 mg SC
- Tinzaparin, 4500 units SC
- Nadroparin, 2850 units SC

Oral direct thrombin inhibitors (dabigatran) and anti-Xa inhibitors (rivaroxaban, apixaban) should be avoided as their safety in pregnancy has not been established.

59.1 THROMBOPROPHYLAXIS FOR CAESAREAN SECTION

All women undergoing CS should be assessed for thromboembolism risk and given appropriate prophylaxis, depending on their risk category. A thromboembolism risk assessment proforma should be completed by the doctor obtaining consent for surgery.

59.2 LOW RISK

- Elective CS
- Uncomplicated pregnancy and no other risk factors

DOI: 10.1201/9781315099897-67

59.2.1 Prophylaxis

- Thromboembolism-deterrent stockings (appropriate size and fitted correctly)
- Early mobilization and hydration

59.3 MODERATE RISK

Women with any one of the following risk factors:

- Age >35 years
- Obesity (>80 kg)
- Parity ≥4
- Gross varicose veins
- Current infection
- Pre-eclampsia
- Immobility before surgery (>4 days)
- Major current illness (e.g. heart or lung disease, cancer, inflammatory bowel disease, nephrotic syndrome, or sickle cell disease)
- Emergency CS in labour
- Excessive blood loss

59.3.1 Prophylaxis

- Thromboembolism-deterrent stockings or intermittent pneumatic compression.
- Early mobilization and hydration.
- Dalteparin (Fragmin) 5000 units SC daily until discharge (other LMWH can be substituted).

59.4 HIGH RISK

- Two or more risk factors from the aforementioned.
- Extended major pelvic or abdominal surgery (e.g. CS or hysterectomy).
- Personal or family history of DVT, pulmonary embolism or thrombophilia.
- Paralysis of lower limbs.
- Antiphospholipid antibody (cardiolipin antibody or lupus anticoagulant).

59.4.1 Prophylaxis

- Thromboembolism-deterrent stockings or pneumatic compression.
- Early mobilization and hydration.
- Dalteparin 5000 units SC daily until the fifth postoperative day, or until fully ambulant if longer.
- Continue with dalteparin or warfarin for 6 weeks post-delivery.

The first dose of dalteparin should be given when the patient returns to the postnatal ward.

59.5 THROMBOPROPHYLAXIS IN VAGINAL DELIVERIES

Many women requiring intrapartum thromboprophylaxis will have been identified antenatally. Some will have been commenced on heparin or aspirin earlier in pregnancy. Check the notes for the regimen prescribed. For others, assess the risk and institute prophylaxis as follows.

59.6 LOW RISK

- Uncomplicated pregnancy

59.6.1 Prophylaxis

- Early mobilization and hydration

59.7 MODERATE RISK

Women with any two of the following risk factors:

- Age >35 years
- Obesity (>80 kg at booking)
- Parity ≥4
- Gross varicose veins
- Current infection
- Pre-eclampsia
- Immobility before delivery (>4 days)
- Major current illness (e.g. heart or lung disease, cancer, inflammatory bowel disease, nephrotic syndrome, or sickle cell disease)
- Labour ≥ 12 hours
- Excessive blood loss

59.7.1 Prophylaxis

- Early mobilization and hydration.
- Thromboembolism-deterrent stockings or pneumatic compression.
- Dalteparin 5000 units SC daily until discharge.

59.8 HIGH RISK

- Three or more risk factors from the aforementioned.
- Extended major pelvic or abdominal surgery (e.g. CS or hysterectomy).
- Personal or family history of DVT, PE or thrombophilia.
- Paralysis of lower limbs.
- Antiphospholipid antibody (cardiolipin antibody or lupus anticoagulant).

59.8.1 Prophylaxis

- Thromboembolism-deterrent stockings or pneumatic compression.
- Early mobilization and hydration.
- Dalteparin 5000 units SC daily until the fifth postoperative day, or until fully ambulant if longer.
- Continue with dalteparin or warfarin for 6 weeks post-delivery.

Dalteparin injection should be commenced within 6 hours of delivery.

59.9 RELATIVE AND ABSOLUTE CONTRAINDICATIONS TO THE USE OF DALTEPARIN

Known bleeding disorder
Active antenatal or postpartum bleeding
Anticipated major haemorrhage (e.g. placenta praevia)
Thrombocytopenia
Acute stroke in previous 4 weeks (haemorrhagic or ischaemic)
Severe renal disease
Severe liver disease
Uncontrolled hypertension

59.10 THE USE OF UNFRACTIONATED HEPARIN (UFH)

Where there is an increased risk of haemorrhage or where regional anaesthetic techniques may be required, UFH may be used in preference to dalteparin because of its shorter half-life and relative ease of reversal. Regional analgesia can be safely given 4 hours after a dose of UFH (12 hours after dalteparin).

If UFH is used after CS, the platelet count should be monitored every 2–3 days from days 4–14 or until heparin is stopped.

59.11 REGIONAL ANALGESIA

Discuss with the anaesthetist if epidural/spinal analgesia is planned (see also later).

Thrombin time should be checked before the administration of an epidural/spinal block.

! Regional analgesia reduces the risk of DVT. General anaesthesia increases the risk of DVT.

! Thromboembolism-deterrent stockings can be harmful if fitted incorrectly.

59.12 REGIONAL ANALGESIA AND DALTEPARIN

59.12.1 Insertion of spinal/epidural block

This must not be done until at least 12 hours after the last dose of *prophylactic* dalteparin.

If the woman has been on *therapeutic* doses of dalteparin, regional techniques should be avoided for at least 24 hours after the last dose.

59.12.2 Removal of epidural catheter

This must not be done until 12 hours after the last dose of dalteparin. After removal of the catheter, wait at least 6 hours before administering the next dose of dalteparin.

Acute venous thromboembolism and pulmonary embolism

60

Unless treatment is strongly contraindicated, any woman with clinical features (see later) of VTE should be commenced on treatment with dalteparin pending the confirmation or exclusion of the diagnosis by objective testing.

60.1 RISK FACTORS

- Obesity
- Immobility
- Grandmultiparity
- Previous DVT
- Dehydration
- Surgical procedures
- APH or PPH
- Pre-eclampsia
- Thrombophilia, inherited or acquired
- Medical conditions such as SLE, sickle cell disease, cancer and inflammatory disorders
- Age >35 years
- Infection
- Operative delivery
- Multiple pregnancy
- Long-distance travel

60.2 CLINICAL FEATURES

- Leg pain, swelling or tenderness
- Chest pain, breathlessness, haemoptysis
- Faintness or collapse
- Pyrexia
- Raised jugular venous pressure

DOI: 10.1201/9781315099897-68

60.3 INITIAL INVESTIGATIONS

- FBC
- U/E and LFT
- Coagulation screen
- D-dimer (interpret with caution, its diagnostic value for VTE in pregnancy is tenuous)

> ! **The D-dimer test is a negative predictive test: in the non-pregnant woman, a low level suggests that there is no VTE, but a high level may be physiological in pregnancy.**

Also, normal D-dimer concentrations have been reported in pregnant women with VTE. Trimester-specific reference intervals for D-dimer in pregnancy have been defined.

Thrombophilia testing in the presence of VTE could give false positive result, as protein C, protein S and antithrombin are consumed in thrombosis.

60.4 SUSPECTED DVT

- Compression or duplex ultrasound scan
- Ultrasound negative and low level of clinical suspicion: discontinue anticoagulant treatment
- Ultrasound negative and high level of clinical suspicion: discontinue anticoagulant treatment but repeat the ultrasound scan on days 3 and 7

60.5 SUSPECTED PE

- Pulse oximetry
- Arterial blood gases
- ECG
- Chest X-ray
- If features of VTE also present, Doppler ultrasound leg studies (bilateral) – if this shows thrombosis, no further investigation required; continue anticoagulant treatment
- V/Q scan or computed tomography pulmonary angiogram (CTPA) – refer to local protocol. If chest X-ray is abnormal, CTPA is preferable to a V/Q scan

Any woman with signs or symptoms suggestive of VTE should undergo diagnostic imaging to confirm or exclude the diagnosis.

If it is not possible to perform diagnostic imaging on the same day, then treatment (see later) should be initiated while awaiting objective diagnosis unless treatment is strongly contraindicated.

60.5.1 Management

- See the algorithms shown in Figures 60.1 and 60.2
- Consult a haematologist
- Apply graduated elastic compression stockings
- Administer anticoagulant treatment (see later)
- For DVT, measure leg circumference daily
- Encourage ambulation

60.6 ANTICOAGULANT THERAPY FOR DVT AND PE

60.6.1 Low-molecular-weight heparin (LMWH)

LMWH (dalteparin, enoxaparin, tinzaparin, bemiparin) is the anticoagulant of choice, barring any special considerations (see later for special circumstances).

The dose is weight-related. Use the weight at booking or the current weight minus 10%.

- Dalteparin 100 IU/kg body weight twice daily, or
- Enoxaparin 1 mg/kg body weight twice daily, or
- Tinzaparin 175 IU/kg

Aim for 4–6 h peak anti-Xa values of 0.6–1.2 IU/mL.

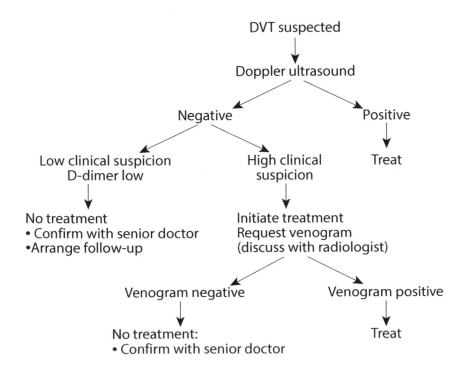

FIGURE 60.1   Algorithm for suspected DVT.

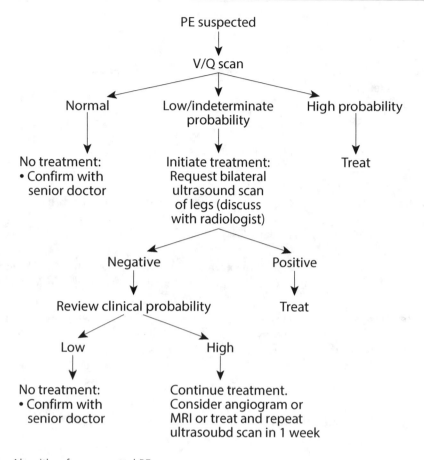

FIGURE 60.2   Algorithm for suspected PE.

! **To work out the dose required: dalteparin 100 IU/kg SC twice daily, up to a maximum of 18 000 units.**

Prescribe and use a prefilled syringe (from a choice of 2500, 5000, 10,000 and 12,500 units) nearest to the calculated requirement.

Do not use less than 10,000 units or more than 18,000 units in 24 hours.

If the body weight is >90 kg or there is renal dysfunction, measure the peak anti-Xa level 3 hours post-injection, aiming for a therapeutic range of 0.6–1.2 IU/mL. Adjust the level of dalteparin as advised by the haematologist, reassessing anti-Xa activity after each dose adjustment.

LMWH maintenance therapy should be discontinued 24 hours prior to planned delivery.

60.6.2 Intravenous unfractionated heparin

This has a shorter half-life than LMWH and is readily reversible with protamine sulphate, so should be considered in the following circumstances:

• Delivery is imminent
• Massive PE

- Floating thrombus on ultrasound scan
- Prosthetic valve
- Renal failure
- Increased risk of bleeding (e.g. as result of coagulopathy, trauma, surgery or peptic ulcer)
- Wound haematoma
- APH or PPH
- Woman at high risk of haemorrhage

Ensure that baseline clotting and platelet count are normal before starting.

- Loading dose: 5000 units IV over 5 minutes.
- Maintenance infusion: Use a preparation of 1000 units/mL. Start at 1 mL/h (i.e. 1000 units/h).

Check the APTT 4–6 hours after the loading dose, aiming for a therapeutic target of 2–2.5 times the average laboratory control value.

Adjust the infusion rate as advised by the haematologist and recheck the APTT every 4–6 hours until the therapeutic ratio is reached. Once the therapeutic ratio is reached, check the APTT at least daily.

In some pregnancies, the therapeutic ratio is difficult to achieve despite high doses of heparin, because fibrinogen and factor VIII levels rise in pregnancy. In such cases, anti-Xa activity should be monitored, aiming for a range of 0.35–0.70 units/mL.

Check the platelet count every 2–3 days from days 4 to 14 or until heparin is stopped.

60.6.3 Contraindications to heparin (including LMWH)

- Active bleeding
- If surgical treatment is to be undertaken (e.g. a caval filter or an embolectomy)
- Previous heparin-induced thrombocytopenia (use danaparoid)
- Previous heparin skin allergy (discuss with the haematologist)

60.7 DURATION OF TREATMENT

Following treatment of the acute phase, anticoagulation should be maintained with LMWH for at least 6 months. In many cases, it will be safe to reduce anticoagulation to a prophylactic dose. Arrange a follow-up appointment with the haematology/coagulation clinic.

60.8 LABOUR AND DELIVERY

A woman on therapeutic anticoagulation should be delivered by planned induction of labour or elective CS at 37–38 weeks. She should be advised that in the event of contractions starting before the day of admission, no further heparin should be self-administered until she has been assessed in hospital.

Women on the standard *prophylactic* dose may await spontaneous onset of labour.

60.9 HIGH RISK WOMAN ON *THERAPEUTIC* LMWH

- Planned delivery at 38–39 weeks.
- Convert LMWH to UFH at least 36 h prior to delivery.
- Stop the UFH infusion 4–6 hours prior to anticipated delivery.
- Check APTT and inform anaesthetist of result.
- *Note*: LMWH can only be partially reversed with protamine sulphate.

60.10 WOMAN ON HIGH DOSE *PROPHYLAXIS*, TWICE-A-DAY REGIMEN

Omit the evening LMWH dose and commence induction or caesarean section the next morning.

Can start regional anaesthesia >24 h after the last dose of LMWH and if no other drugs with impairment of coagulation are used.

60.11 INDUCTION OF LABOUR

- Omit any morning dose of dalteparin on the day of induction.
- On admission: FBC, coagulation profile, anti-Xa and group-and-save.
- Inform the haematologist.
- Dalteparin 5000 units daily (i.e. a prophylactic dose) should be given on admission and continued until the woman has delivered.
- Apply thromboembolism-deterrent stockings.
- There should be active management of the third stage.
- Give a Syntocinon (oxytocin) infusion 40 units in 500 mL Hartmann's solution or 0.9% saline for 4 hours post-delivery.
- The therapeutic regimen should be resumed following delivery.

60.12 ELECTIVE CAESAREAN SECTION

- Omit any morning dose of dalteparin on the day of operation.
- On admission: FBC, coagulation profile, anti-Xa and group-and-save.
- Inform the haematologist.
- Give dalteparin 5000 units SC 3 hours postoperative, or 4 hours after removal of the epidural catheter.
- Consider placing a wound drain.
- Use staples or interrupted sutures for skin.
- Give a Syntocinon infusion 40 units in 500 mL Hartmann's solution or 0.9% saline for 4 hours post-delivery.

- The therapeutic regimen should be resumed the evening after surgery.
- Apply thromboembolism-deterrent stockings.

60.13 THIRD STAGE OF LABOUR

Administer 2 IU oxytocin over 5 min.

Followed by infusion: 10 U of oxytocin in 500 mL of normal saline given IV at 36 mL/h for 4 h (12 mU/min)]

60.14 EPIDURAL OR SPINAL ANAESTHESIA

This should be discussed with the woman before induction of labour or CS.

- If the woman is on a therapeutic dose of LMWH, a regional block should not be used until at least 24 hours after the last dose.
- If the woman is on a prophylactic dose (this should be the case if the aforementioned protocol for induction and elective CS has been followed), a regional block should not be used until at least 12 hours after the last dose.

LMWH should not be given for at least 6 hours after the epidural catheter has been removed. The cannula should not be removed within 12 hours of the most recent injection.

60.15 POSTPARTUM ANTICOAGULATION

Anticoagulation should be continued for at least 6 weeks. If the woman opts for an oral anticoagulant (warfarin), this can be started on the day following delivery. Breastfeeding is not a contraindication to warfarin.

Major haemoglobinopathy

61

The major haemoglobinopathies are sickle cell disease (SCD) and thalassaemia. These should be excluded in women of African, Asian or Mediterranean origin. Major haemoglobinopathy should be suspected when there is anaemia in the absence of bleeding in a woman from any of these populations (but haemoglobinopathy is not exclusive to them).

Pregnant women with SCD are more likely to experience pre-eclampsia, venous thromboembolism, infections, fetal growth restriction, preterm delivery, stillbirth and maternal mortality.

A sickle cell crisis may be precipitated or exacerbated by hypoxia/acidosis, dehydration and infection.

61.1 PRINCIPLES OF MANAGEMENT IN LABOUR

- Avoid dehydration, infection, acidosis, hypoxia and prolonged labour
- Liaise with the haematologist and the blood transfusion laboratory
- Inform the anaesthetist and paediatrician on admission
- Vaginal birth not contraindicated. Discuss birth positions if there is a history of hip replacement
- Any fever should be taken seriously
- If administering a Syntocinon (oxytocin) drip, avoid fluid overload
- In cases of PROM, labour should be induced to minimize the risk of chorioamnionitis
- Do not give an iron supplement
- Encourage ambulation

61.2 ACTION PLAN

- Record BP and do a urinalysis on admission
- Check FBC, U/E, LFT, urates, creatinine and blood gases on admission
- Establish IV access
- Cross-match 4 units of blood
- Initiate continuous CTG monitoring
- Set up pulse oximetry
- Administer oxygen
- Provide a liberal oral fluid intake or judicious use of IV fluids
- Give antibiotic cover – penicillin
- Recommend epidural analgesia, especially where operative delivery is anticipated, but:
  - Avoid overload when giving IV fluid before epidural
  - Use elastic stockings and leg elevation to avoid hypotension and venous pooling in the legs

DOI: 10.1201/9781315099897-69

- Watch for signs of PE
- Consider thromboembolism prophylaxis
- There should be active management of the third stage
- Take cord blood for FBC and haemoglobin electrophoresis

61.3 SICKLE CELL CRISIS

61.3.1 Bone pain crisis (vaso-occlusive crisis)

- Fever
- Painful limbs, chest and abdomen
- Tender bones and abdomen

61.3.2 Acute chest syndrome

- Signs and symptoms of lower respiratory tract disease (breathlessness, cough, wheezing, etc.)
- ± fever

61.3.3 Sequestration (rbcs and platelets are sequestered in the spleen)

- Bone pain
- Abdominal pain, fever
- Hepatomegaly
- Splenomegaly
- Falling [Hb] but rising reticulocyte count and circulating nucleated rbcs

61.3.4 Aplastic crisis (precipitated by parvovirus B19)

- Fever
- Dyspnoea
- Pallor
- Low [Hb]
- Low reticulocyte count

61.4 ACTION PLAN

- Involve the haematologist
- Maintain airway oxygen via a facemask, 15 L/min
- Assess pulse and BP
- Monitor O_2 saturation

- ECG
- Establish IV access: FBC, U/E, reticulocyte count and LFT
- Check arterial blood gases
- Do a sepsis screen: blood culture and a midstream specimen of urine for bacteriology
- Do a chest X-ray if there are chest symptoms
- Rehydrate with Hartmann's solution or 0.9% saline
- Monitor fluid input and urine output
- Administer parenteral analgesia. Consider opioid administration by patient-controlled analgesia (PCA). Pethidine should not be used because of the associated risk of seizures
- Administer IV antibiotics
- Treat the cause of the crisis if identified
- Cross-match 4 units of blood (the laboratory must be informed that the woman has sickle cell disease)
- Give a transfusion as required (packed cells) – discuss with the haematologist. A transfusion is not usually required if [Hb] ≥ 6 g/dL

61.4.1 May need urgent exchange transfusion

61.4.1.1 Obtain her transfusion history

Side effects of transfusion in patients with sickle cell disease include alloimmunization, autoimmunization, iron overload, haemolysis and hyperviscosity. These should be discussed with the haematologist.

Inherited coagulation disorders

62

Haemophilia and von Willebrand disease

Coagulation disorders can be inherited or acquired:

- **Inherited**: haemophilia, von Willebrand disease, factor XI deficiency and other rare disorders.
- **Acquired**: gestational thrombocytopenia and immune thrombocytopenic purpura (ITP, Chapter 63).

62.1 HAEMOPHILIA

- Haemophilia A is due to a deficiency of factor VIII. The partial thromboplastin time (PTT) is usually prolonged. The platelet count, bleeding time and prothrombin time (PT) are normal.
- Normal levels of FVIII: 50%–150%.
- Haemophilia B is due to deficiency of factor IX. The prothrombin time is usually prolonged.
- Both are X-linked recessive disorders. The sex of the fetus may not be known, so cases should be managed on the presumption that the fetus is male.
- Most carriers do not have bleeding problems, but a small number tend to bleed, owing to low clotting factor levels.
- Haemophilia A can be treated with factor VIII concentrates, cryoprecipitate and fresh frozen plasma.
- Cryoprecipitate does not contain adequate concentration of factor IX so is not useful for treatment of haemophilia B. Treat with factor IX concentrates.
- Haemophilia C is due to a lack of coagulation factor XI. It has been observed mostly in persons of Ashkenazi Jewish ancestry.
- Types of clotting factor infusion: plasma-derived (made from human plasma) and recombinant (made with DNA technology).
- The new drug emicizumab is effective for haemophilia A but there are no clinical studies of its use in pregnant women.

DOI: 10.1201/9781315099897-70

62.2 VON WILLEBRAND DISEASE

This is a group of autosomally inherited disorders characterized by reduced synthesis of von Willebrand factor (vWF) or by structural or functional defects in this factor.

vWF is a protein involved in platelet adhesion. Apart from being essential for normal platelet function, it acts as a carrier for factor VIII, so patients with von Willebrand disease usually have prolonged bleeding time and reduced factor VIII procoagulant activity (VIII:C) activity.

Von Willebrand disease is classified into three types:

- Type 1, there is a partial deficiency in the production of vWF, but its structure and function are normal;
- Type 2 (of which there are a few subtypes), the amount of vWF produced may be normal, but the structure and function are abnormal;
- Type 3, there is total or near total deficiency in vWF.
- Bleeding is more frequent and more severe in types 2 and 3.

Type 1 is autosomal dominant, type 2 is usually autosomal dominant (rarely autosomal recessive) and type 3 is autosomal recessive.

- The incidence of primary PPH is high, and the incidence of secondary PPH is even higher. In severe cases, discuss with the haematologist regarding treatment with desmopressin acetate (DDAVP) or vWF concentrate (plasma-derived or recombinant).
  DDAVP causes release of factor VIII from endothelial cells and is effective in Type 1. Its side effects include mild tachycardia, flushing and headache. Urine output and fluid balance should be monitored to avoid hyponatremia.
- Tranexamic acid 1 g three times daily should be given immediately following delivery and continued for 5 days. Secondary PPH may also be treated with tranexamic acid.

62.3 ACTION PLAN

- Check notes for the plan agreed with the consultant haematologist
- Ascertain the availability of blood products as required
- FBC
- Do coagulation tests
- Check clotting factor levels (factor VIIIc in haemophilia A and factor IX in haemophilia B)
  If levels are <50 IU/dL, transfuse with recombinant factor VIII or IX and recheck 30 minutes after transfusion
- Group-and-save
- Avoid IM injections
- Avoid NSAIDs
- Epidural analgesia may be given, provided that the coagulation screen is normal and the platelet count is >100 × 10^9/L. Epidural analgesia is also considered safe if clotting factor levels are >50 IU/dL
- Repeat the coagulation screen before removing the epidural catheter
- Avoid the use of FSE and FBS, since an affected fetus may bleed (the sex of the unborn baby is not usually known)

- Make early recourse to CS in cases of slow progress
- Avoid vacuum-assisted delivery (a low forceps delivery may be performed and is preferable to a traumatic CS delivery)
- If CS or instrumental delivery is required, ensure that clotting factor levels are >50 IU/L. If they are <50 IU/L, transfuse with recombinant factor VIII or IX, as appropriate
- Anticipate PPH
- Factor VIII and factor IX fall rapidly after delivery. Post-delivery, ensure that clotting factor activity is >50 IU/dL for 5 days, to minimize the risk of PPH

In type 1 VWD, if FVIII:C and/or VWF <30 U/dL, administer DDAVP after umbilical clamping and continue for 3–4 days postpartum.

62.4 THE NEONATE

- Obtain cord blood in a citrated bottle from all male babies for investigation.
- Give the neonate oral vitamin K.
- Perform a cranial ultrasound scan if there is any suggestion of possible intracranial bleed (e.g. poor feeding, lethargy or vomiting).
- Inform the GP so that the neonate's immunizations are given subcutaneously or intradermally.

Immune thrombocytopenic purpura

63

Immune thrombocytopenic purpura (ITP) is a condition in which platelets are destroyed prematurely by antiplatelet antibodies. There is no diagnostic test – the condition is diagnosed by exclusion of other causes of thrombocytopenia. The platelet count is persistently low (<100 × 10^9/L), but the FBC, blood film, PT and APTT are normal. Tests for antiplatelet antibodies are non-specific and do not distinguish ITP from gestational thrombocytopenia. Bone marrow biopsy may be needed for diagnosis.

When seen on the delivery suite, the woman will fall into one of the following groups, depending on what treatment she has received:

- **Asymptomatic and with platelet count >50 × 10^9/L**: requires no treatment.
- **Been on prednisolone for maintenance of platelet count**: give hydrocortisone 100 mg IV every 8 hours to cover labour and delivery (because of inhibition of the pituitary–adrenal axis): watch for hyperglycaemia.
- **IV immunoglobulin given just before induction of labour or CS**: watch for side effects of headache, nausea, alopecia and abnormal LFT.

63.1 DIFFERENTIAL DIAGNOSES OF THROMBOCYTOPENIA IN PREGNANCY

- Gestational thrombocytopenia
- Pre-eclampsia; HELLP
- Idiopathic thrombocytopenic purpura
- Systemic lupus erythematosus (SLE)
- Antiphospholipid syndrome
- Disseminated intravascular coagulation (DIC)
- Thrombotic thrombocytopenic purpura
- Other systemic disorder, e.g. viral infection, haemolytic uremic syndrome

63.2 ACTION PLAN

- Check notes for the plan agreed with the consultant haematologist
- FBC

DOI: 10.1201/9781315099897-71

- LFT
- Obtain a coagulation profile
- Check clotting factor levels
- Confirm availability and access to platelets for transfusion
- Alert paediatricians (the baby is at risk of thrombocytopenia, which carries a risk of intracranial haemorrhage)
- Avoid intramuscular injection of pethidine
- Discuss pain relief with the consultant anaesthetist
- Epidural is not contraindicated if:
  - FBC is normal
  - the coagulation profile is normal
  - clotting factor levels are >50 IU/L during the third trimester
- Platelet count >80,000/μl. Hematoma following neuroaxial anaesthesia is rare above this level
- Check factor levels before removing the epidural catheter
- Obtain an anticoagulated cord blood sample and send it immediately to the haemophilia laboratory

To rapidly increase the platelet count: intravenous immunoglobulin (IVIg) 2 gm/kg over 2–5 days.

63.3 MODE OF DELIVERY

The mode of delivery in cases of ITP remains a subject of debate. In each case, it should be decided by the consultant obstetrician and consultant haematologist, with the consent of the woman. If the platelet count is $<50 \times 10^9$/L, then platelet transfusion and CS may decrease the risk of intracranial haemorrhage in the neonate.

Avoid the use of FSE and vacuum-assisted delivery.

63.4 THE NEONATE

Antiplatelet antibodies may cross the placenta, causing fetal thrombocytopenia. This may manifest as purpura, haematuria or intracranial haemorrhage. Neither prednisolone therapy nor IV immunoglobulin given to the mother can prevent fetal thrombocytopenia.

The risk of bleeding is low if the fetus has a platelet count of $>50 \times 10^9$/L, but obtaining a sample of fetal blood is risky and requires special skills.

63.5 POSTNATAL CARE

- Give vitamin K orally.
- Do serial platelet counts at birth and during the first week postpartum.
- Routine immunizations should be given subcutaneously or intradermally.
- Consider hepatitis B immunization.

Thrombophilia

64

Thrombophilia is an abnormality of haemostasis predisposing to thrombosis. It may be:

- **Hereditary**:
    - Activated protein C resistance (associated with factor V Leiden mutation)
    - Protein C deficiency
    - Protein S deficiency
    - Antithrombin deficiency
    - Prothrombin gene mutation
- **Acquired**:
    - Antiphospholipid syndrome
    - Acquired activated protein C resistance
    - Polycythaemia
    - Other conditions (e.g. malignancy)

Hyperhomocysteinaemia is a thrombophilia with genetic and acquired origins.

About 50% of thromboembolic events in pregnancy occur in women with an identifiable thrombophilia. Women with thrombophilia are also at increased risk of stillbirth, IUGR and pre-eclampsia.

64.1 MANAGEMENT IN LABOUR

Most women with known thrombophilia will have been commenced on anticoagulant treatment antenatally. See peripartum management of anticoagulant therapy in Chapter 60.

- Check the notes for the management plan as outlined by the consultant obstetrician or haematologist
- Discontinue heparin/LMWH if in labour or before induction of labour
- FBC
- Do a coagulation screen: APTT, PT and anti-Xa assay (if available)
- Watch for pre-eclampsia developing in labour

64.2 EPIDURAL ANALGESIA

This may be considered if:

- Heparin/LMWH has not been given in the preceding 6 hours.
- The coagulation screen is normal.
- The platelet count is >100×10^9/L.

DOI: 10.1201/9781315099897-72

64.3 POSTPARTUM

- Resume anticoagulant prophylaxis 12 hours after delivery (unless bleeding is more than lochial loss).

  Women with previous VTE associated with antithrombin deficiency or the antiphospholipid syndrome (APS) and those with recurrent VTE should be offered thromboprophylaxis with higher dose LMWH (either 50%, 75% or full treatment dose) antenatally and for 6 weeks postpartum or until returned to oral anticoagulant therapy after delivery.
- Continue anticoagulant prophylaxis for 3 months.
- Oral anticoagulants may be started within the first 2 days, and heparin/LMWH should be withdrawn when the International Normalized Ratio (INR) has been within the therapeutic range for 3 days.
- In cases of heritable thrombophilia, inform the parents of the risk of autosomal transmission.

Gestational thrombocytopenia

65

This is a mild reduction in platelet count occurring in the second or third trimester, with no bleeding problems for mother or baby. The platelet count is usually in the range $100-150 \times 10^9/L$ and reverts to normal after pregnancy.

- Vaginal delivery is safe.
- Regional analgesia is safe.
- Platelet count returns to normal 2–12 weeks after delivery.

DOI: 10.1201/9781315099897-73

Antepartum haemorrhage

66

Antepartum haemorrhage (APH) is defined formally as bleeding from the genital tract after 24 weeks' gestation. In practice, vaginal bleeding that occurs after a woman has had a normal fetal anatomy scan is managed as APH.

66.1 RCOG CLASSIFICATION OF APH

- Spotting – staining, streaking or blood spotting noted on underwear or sanitary protection.
- Minor haemorrhage – blood loss less than 50 mL that has settled.
- Major haemorrhage – blood loss of 50–1000 mL, with no signs of clinical shock.
- Massive haemorrhage – blood loss greater than 1000 mL and/or signs of clinical shock.

66.2 DIFFERENTIAL DIAGNOSES

APH is not a diagnosis but an observation. The differential diagnoses are:

- Placenta praevia (Chapter 67)
- Placental abruption (concealed bleeding could be more significant than revealed loss)
- Bleeding from the cervix (ectopy, polyp, carcinoma, etc.)
- Vasa praevia

66.3 PLACENTAL ABRUPTION

There are three grades of placental abruption:

- Grade 1. Small amount of vaginal bleeding and some uterine contractions but no signs of fetal distress or low blood pressure in the mother.
- Grade 2. Mild to medium amount of bleeding and uterine contractions. The baby's heart rate shows signs of distress and the mother's pulse rate may be elevated.
- Grade 3. Medium to severe bleeding (sometimes revealed, other times concealed within the womb). Also, unrelenting uterine contractions, abdominal pain, low blood pressure, and the death of the baby.

DOI: 10.1201/9781315099897-74

66.4 ASSESSMENT

- Assess blood loss.
- Check BP, pulse and respiration.
- If the woman is in shock: airway, breathing, circulation.
- Exclude abdominal pain and contractions.
- Exclude placenta praevia before performing a digital vaginal examination.

! Note that abruption of a posterior placenta may present as back pain.

66.5 MINOR APH (MINIMAL LOSS, <50 ML ON ADMISSION)

- Check scan reports for placental site (but note that scans can be wrong)
- Perform a speculum examination
- FBC, group-and-save; do a Kleihauer test if the woman is Rh-negative
- CTG
- If the woman is Rh-negative, give anti-D 1000 units IM
- Transfer to the ward if there is no major bleeding, uterine tenderness or fetal distress

66.6 MAJOR APH (SIGNIFICANT BLEEDING, 50–1000 ML BUT NOT IN SHOCK)

- Insert an IV line (14G). Crystalloid infusion.
- FBC, U/E, clotting, cross-match 4 units; do a Kleihauer test if the woman is Rh-negative.
- Catheterize and monitor urine output.
- Set up an intensive monitoring chart.
- Inform the anaesthetist and neonatal unit.
- Inform the consultant: a decision must be made regarding the mode and timing of delivery.
- If the woman is Rh-negative and delivery is not imminent, give anti-D 1000 units IM.
- Monitor on the delivery suite for up to 12 hours post-delivery.

66.7 MASSIVE APH (ESTIMATED LOSS >1000 ML AND/OR SIGNS OF CLINICAL SHOCK)

- Call for a senior obstetrician, anaesthetist, theatre team and porters. Alert the blood bank and haematology laboratory
- Administer oxygen by mask: 10–15 L/min

- Keep the woman warm
- Left lateral tilt
- Insert two IV lines with 14G, or larger, cannulas
- Catheterize and monitor urine output hourly
- ECG
- Set up pulse oximetry
- Initiate serial BP recording
- Consider an arterial line and CVP. This is likely to be required if blood loss is more than 1500 mL or if the woman is to be taken to theatre

> ! 'Failure to use [invasive] monitoring in the treatment of major obstetric haemorrhage is substandard care.'
>
> Thomas TA, Cooper GM. Anaesthesia. In: Lewis G, ed. *Why Mothers Die 1997–1999.*
> *The Confidential Enquiries into Maternal Deaths in the United Kingdom.*
> London: RCOG Press, 2001:143

The clinical situation may have changed by the time blood results are available, so treat the patient, not the results.

- FBC, PT, APTT, FDP and fibrinogen.
- Urgently cross-match 6 units of blood.
- Give plasma substitutes: Haemaccel or Gelofusine 2000 mL immediately.
- Transfuse cross-matched blood if available.
- If cross-matched blood is not available immediately, use:
  - Unmatched blood (patient's group), which is usually available within 15 minutes
  - Group O negative blood (emergency stock) – if blood is needed immediately.
- **Before using uncross-matched blood, always:**
  - **Discuss with the laboratory.**
  - **Obtain the woman's blood sample for tests listed earlier.**
- Use 4 units FFP for every 6 units of packed cells or if PT and APPT are >1.5 × control.
- Transfuse platelets concentrates if platelet count <50 × 109/l.

Platelet transfusion is usually needed with 1.5–2 times blood volume replacement.

- Transfuse cryoprecipitate if fibrinogen <1 g/l.

Further transfusion of coagulation factors may be required.

> ! Blood-warming equipment should be used.

- Continuous CTG monitoring.
- Record blood loss: weigh soaked linen.
- If CTG is normal and bleeding has settled, perform an ultrasound scan. A scan is also indicated if fetal heart tones are not detected.
- Consider early transfer to ITU/HDU.

'A standing agreement between the haematologists and obstetricians over the issue of platelets, FFP and cryoprecipitate reduces the number of phone calls required and speeds response. Coagulation monitoring will help to assess the adequacy of the coagulation support and guide the selection of components but should not delay the initial issue of FFP or cryoprecipitate.'

Blood Transfusion Services of the United Kingdom. Obstetric haemorrhage.
In: McClelland DBL, ed. Handbook of Transfusion Medicine, 3rd edn.
London: The Stationery Office, 2001:80

66.8 DELIVERY

- The senior obstetrician makes the decision regarding urgency and mode of delivery.
- If fetal death has occurred, counsel for vaginal birth.
- There should be active management of the third stage of labour.
- APH predisposes to PPH, so a Syntocinon (oxytocin) infusion (40 units in 500 mL Hartmann's solution or 0.9% saline) should be commenced in the third stage of labour and continued for 4 hours post-delivery.

Major placenta praevia

67

- Deliver only in a unit equipped to deal with massive haemorrhage.
- Uncomplicated placenta praevia – deliver at 36–37 weeks.
- Placenta praevia with history of bleeding – deliver at 34–26 weeks.
- If she presents with preterm contractions and not requiring immediate delivery, offer tocolysis and antental corticosteroids.
- Vaginal delivery is contraindicated if the placenta encroaches within 2 cm of the internal os.
- Elective or emergency CS for major placenta praevia should be performed only by a consultant obstetrician or by an experienced obstetrician with the consultant in attendance.
- At CS, do not cut through the placenta. On incising the myometrium, insinuate a hand through the incision to reach and rupture the amniotic sac above the placenta while delivering the baby simultaneously.

67.1 ACTION PLAN

- FBC
- Discuss blood transfusion
- Cross-match 4–6 units of blood
- Note whether she has atypical antibodies
- Liaise with interventional radiologist
- In cases of anterior placenta praevia in a scarred uterus (i.e. previous CS), the woman should be informed of the possibility of placenta accreta
- Consent should be obtained for a hysterectomy to be performed in the event of uncontrollable bleeding
- Arrange for cell salvage (see next section)
- Anticipate PPH: commence Syntocinon (oxytocin) infusion (40 units in 500 mL Hartmann's solution or 0.9% saline) immediately after delivery of the baby

! In the event of massive haemorrhage, manage as outlined.

If bleeding is not controlled by pharmacological and conservative surgical interventions, do not delay in proceeding to hysterectomy.

DOI: 10.1201/9781315099897-75

67.2 CELL SALVAGE

Consider this if:

- There is a high risk of massive bleeding (>1000mL) at surgery, e.g. placental abruption, placenta praevia, placenta accreta spectrum, large uterine fibroids.
- Low pre-operative haemoglobin.
- Rare blood group/multiple antibodies.
- She objects to receiving allogeneic blood.

Sickle cell disease and heparin-induced thrombocytopenia are relative contraindications.

67.2.1 Action plan

- Obtain consent
- Ensure there are no contaminants in the operating field (e.g. Surgicel and Floseal)
- No cases of amniotic fluid embolism from reinfusion have been reported
- If she is Rh(D)-negative, nonsensitized and has received salvaged red cells and the baby is confirmed to be Rh(D)-positive (or unknown), administer a minimum of 1500 IU anti-D immunoglobulin
- To confirm if more anti-D is needed, obtain her blood sample for estimation of fetomaternal haemorrhage 30–40 minutes after reinfusion of salvaged red cells
- Administration of anti-D should occur within 72 hours of delivery
- Report any adverse event associated with reinfusion

CLINICAL SAFETY INCIDENT FROM 2021 SHOT ANNUAL REPORT:

Failure to inform the transfusion laboratory of cell salvage reinfusion

An Rh(D)-negative mother delivered by emergency caesarean section, and cell salvage was used during the procedure.

The transfusion laboratory was not informed that cell salvage had been used for this patient.

The patient received 515 mL of salvaged blood and baby was D-positive so she should have been given 1500 IU anti-D immunoglobulin (Ig). However, because the transfusion laboratory staff were unaware that cell salvage had been used, only 500 IU anti-D Ig was issued to the patient. This was discovered retrospectively by the transfusion practitioner after receiving the cell salvage data collection form.

Placenta accreta spectrum

68

Morbidly adherent placenta which, depending on degree of myometrial invasion, may be placenta increta, placenta percreta or placenta accreta.

Anticipate placenta accreta spectrum if there is a history of any of the following:

- Accreta in a previous pregnancy
- Previous caesarean delivery
- Any surgical operation on the uterus
- Asherman syndrome
- Placenta praevia
- Caesarean scar pregnancy

Placenta praevia is present in >80% of cases.

If there is a combination of previous caesarean section and placenta praevia in the current pregnancy, treat as placenta accreta spectrum until proven otherwise.

68.1 INVESTIGATION

- Ultrasound scan (USS). Very high sensitivity and specificity but note that the absence of ultrasound findings does not preclude a diagnosis of placenta accreta spectrum.
- MR scan, if necessary, to assess the depth of invasion.

68.2 DELIVERY

Planned delivery at 35–36 + 0 weeks, by a multidisciplinary team in a unit with appropriate expertise and facilities.

Make prearrangements in case an emergency delivery is needed (various obstetric indications).

Discuss the following with the woman:

- Role and risk/benefits of interventional radiology
- Massive obstetric haemorrhage
- Blood transfusion
- Risk of urinary tract injury
- Risk of hysterectomy

DOI: 10.1201/9781315099897-76

- Administer prophylactic steroids for fetal lung maturity
- Alert the urologist
- Liaise with interventional radiologist
- Liaise with blood bank
- Administer intravenous tranexamic acid at the commencement of surgery
- The surgical approach with the least probability of massive haemorrhage is caesarean section followed immediately by hysterectomy, with the placenta left in its implantation site. Confirm that the placenta has not separated before proceeding to remove the uterus
- If the woman wishes to preserve her uterus and accepts the attendant risks, the placenta will be removed after delivery of the baby at caesarean section. Following removal of the placenta, insert a Bakri balloon

There is no room for heroics here; rather proceed to hysterectomy if bleeding is not arrested promptly.

- Closing the abdomen after caesarean section, with the placenta retained in situ and left to autolyse ('expectant management') is in theory an alternative approach but is not recommended in this handbook.
- Activate the massive haemorrhage protocol.
- Offer tranexamic acid 1 g intravenously within 3 hours of birth.

Retained placenta

69

By definition, 'retained placenta' occurs when the placenta has shown no signs of separation after 20 minutes of delivery of the baby (60 minutes if the third stage has been managed physiologically).

The following plan also applies when the placenta has been delivered but there are missing cotyledons.

> ! In the case of a scarred uterus, beware of placenta accreta. Obtain consent for possible blood transfusion and hysterectomy before proceeding to manual removal.

In some cases of retained placenta, the placenta will separate following injection of a mixture of Syntocinon (oxytocin) 50 units and 30 mL 0.9% saline into the umbilical vein.

69.1 ACTION PLAN

- Inform the registrar.
- Ensure that the bladder is empty.
- Insert an IV line (14G or larger).
- Give a Syntocinon infusion 40 units in 500 mL Hartmann's solution or 0.9% saline.
- Group-and-save (cross-match if bleeding is >500 mL).
- Monitor pulse, BP and blood loss.
- Counsel the woman regarding the possibility of placenta accreta.
- Remove the retained placenta manually in theatre under spinal or epidural analgesia. (A general anaesthetic is preferable only if the patient is shocked or bleeding heavily.)
- If the placenta is morbidly adherent, call the consultant immediately.
- Continue Syntocinon infusion for 4 hours after manual removal.
- Give IV co-amoxiclav (Augmentin) or cefuroxime/metronidazole as a bolus.
- If uterine inversion occurs during the process of manual removal, then reduce the inversion before any further attempt at removing the placenta. Call the consultant immediately. See also Chapter 87 (Uterine inversion).

DOI: 10.1201/9781315099897-77

Postpartum haemorrhage

70

> ! Only two-thirds of all postpartum haemorrhages (PPH) occur in women with known risk factors.

> ! At CS, blood loss is likely to be higher if the placenta is removed manually than if it were removed by cord traction.

70.1 ACTION PLAN

- Summon help

For major haemorrhage:

- Call the team leader, obstetricians, anaesthetist, porter and other members of the theatre team
- Alert the blood bank and haematologist
- Nominate a recorder
- Assess airway, breathing and circulation
- Give uterine massage
- Administer oxygen by mask
- Keep her warm
- Catheterize and monitor urine output
- Assess blood loss
- Insert two wide-bore IV cannulae (14G or larger)
- FBC
- Urea and electrolytes
- LFT
- Clotting profile
- Urgent cross-match 6 units
- Give oxytocic drugs, as may be required, in the following order
- Syntocinon (oxytocin) 10 units IM bolus
- Syntocinon infusion 40 units in 500 mL Hartmann's solution
- ergometrine 0.5 mg IV (an antiemetic may be given simultaneously)
- carboprost (Hemabate) 0.25 mg IM, repeated every 15 minutes, up to eight doses (maximum dose 2 mg)

DOI: 10.1201/9781315099897-78

☐ Administer *intravenous* tranexamic acid (TXA).

This must be given within 3 hours of birth, in all cases of PPH, regardless of cause.
Dose: 1 g in 10 mL (100 mg/mL) IV at 1 mL per minute, i.e. administered over 10 minutes.

☐ Give a second dose of 1 g IV if bleeding continues after 30 minutes
☐ Infuse plasma substitutes: IV Haemaccel or Gelofusine 2 L immediately
☐ Serial BP monitoring
☐ Pulse oximetry
☐ Arterial line/CVP monitoring

> ! 'Failure to use [invasive monitoring] in the treatment of major obstetric haemorrhage is substandard care.'
>
> *Thomas TA, Cooper GM. Anaesthesia. In: Lewis G, ed. Why Mothers Die 1997–1999:*
> *The Confidential Enquiries into Maternal Deaths in the United Kingdom. London:*
> *RCOG Press, 2001:143*

☐ Record pulse rate, BP, O$_2$ saturation, CVP and other observations on a high-dependency chart and record the early warning score.
☐ Diagnose and treat the source of bleeding – 'the four Ts':
  ☐ **T**one
  ☐ **T**rauma
  ☐ **T**issue (placenta)
  ☐ **T**hrombin (clotting)
☐ The frequency of repeat blood tests is determined by the clinical situation, but in major bleeding this is usually every 4 hours until stable.
☐ Estimate the blood loss: weigh soaked linen and swabs.
☐ Consider early transfer to HDU or ITU.

70.2 RETAINED PLACENTA

Proceed immediately to manual removal.

70.3 UTERINE ATONY

Give an oxytocic regimen as mentioned earlier.

Also consider the use of a Bakri or Sengstaken–Blakemore tube. Before using the tube, ensure that there are no retained products of conception. Inflate the balloon with sterile fluid (see product label for maximum volume). Leave for 24 hours, and then deflate. The Bakri balloon has an inner lumen which enables assessment of ongoing blood loss.

Consider inserting a compression suture (see description of technique later).

70.4 GENITAL TRACT TRAUMA OR UNDIAGNOSED BLEEDING

Proceed to EUA. Counsel for laparotomy and possible hysterectomy. Good light and good assistance are essential for EUA.

70.5 COAGULOPATHY

Manage in collaboration with a haematologist. The clinical situation may have changed by the time blood results are available, so treat the patient, not the results. Treat coagulation defects as advised by the haematologist. See also 'Transfusion of blood products' next.

! **Take care**: in the rush to get things done, a blood specimen is sometimes sent to the laboratory either unlabelled or with incorrect identity.

70.6 TRANSFUSION OF BLOOD PRODUCTS

- Transfuse cross-matched blood if available.
- If cross-matched blood is not available immediately, use:
  - Unmatched blood (patient's group), which is usually available within 15 minutes
  - Group O negative blood (emergency stock) – if blood is needed immediately (i.e. in a life-threatening situation).

Before using uncross-matched blood, always:
- Discuss with the laboratory.
- Obtain the woman's blood sample for the tests listed earlier.
- Use blood-warming equipment.
- Infuse with a pressure bag.

70.6.1 Fresh frozen plasma (FFP)

Transfusion of FFP is usually required if blood loss/replacement approaches the estimated blood volume of the woman. After 6 units of red blood cells, infuse FFP 12–15 mL/kg.

Aim for prothrombin time (PT) and activated partial thromboplastin time (APTT) ratios of not less than 1.5 × normal.

70.6.2 Platelets

- Transfuse if platelet count $<80 \times 10^9/l$.
- Platelet transfusion is usually needed with 1.5–2 times blood volume replacement.
- If she is Rh(D)-negative, give Rh(D)-negative platelets.

70.6.3 Cryoprecipitate

Cryoprecipitate is likely to be needed if the fibrinogen level is abnormally low. Target: plasma fibrinogen >1.5–2 g/l.

70.7 COMPRESSION SUTURE

70.7.1 B-Lynch suture

A large Mayo needle with absorbable suture is used to enter and exit the uterine cavity through a hysterotomy incision and looped over the fundus as shown in Figure 70.1.

The suture should then be pulled tight. Once the suture has been double-looped as shown, the loose ends are tied down securely to compress the uterus.

70.7.2 Hayman suture

A modification of the B-Lynch suture that is performed without a hysterotomy.

Vertical compression sutures (2–4) are placed, but in contrast to the B-Lynch technique, these sutures pass directly from the anterior uterine wall to the posterior uterine wall.

A transverse suture is placed if needed to control bleeding from the lower uterine segment.

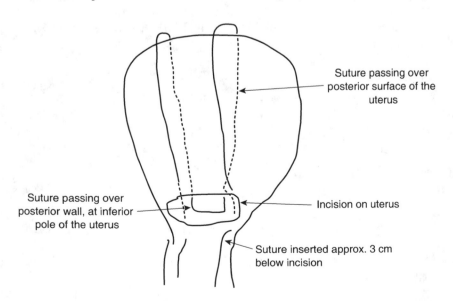

FIGURE 70.1   The B-Lynch compression suture.

70.8 WHERE COULD THINGS GO WRONG?

- Failure to anticipate high-risk patients.
- Being falsely reassured by a systolic BP >100 mmHg. Usually, systolic pressure does not fall until a minimum of 1.5 L has been lost.
- Inadequate blood transfusion or excessive use of fluids.
- Delay between ordering of blood products and their arrival.
- Failure to detect early DIC and respond appropriately.
- Lack of involvement of senior staff at an early stage.
- Delay in resort to surgical treatment.

70.9 DOCUMENTATION

The nature, time and outcome of any intervention should be documented (free text or proforma). See proforma designed by the author (Figure 70.2).

POSTPARTUM HAEMORRHAGE (PPH) PROFORMA

Patient identification

Stick label here or write name, hospital number and date of birth

Baby delivered at ....(time)

Transferred to operating room?

No ☐ Yes ☐ Time ....

Initial observations and management

BP.................. HR ....
  O₂ sat............ MEWS ....

Uterine massage ☐

Bimanual compression ☐

Catheterised Yes ☐ No ☐

Urometer Yes ☐ No ☐

IV access (large bore) ☐

Bloods sent:

FBC ☐ U+E ☐ Coag ☐ G+S ☐

X-match ☐ ....units

Oxygen given ☐

IV fluids given ☐ ....

Blood transfusion

Estimated blood loss ....mL

Swabs weighed? Yes ☐ No ☐

Pre-delivery Hb ....

Needs transfusion? Yes ☐ No ☐

Blood requested ☐ Time? ....

How many units given initially? ....

Time commenced...................

Type? (O-Neg, Group specific) ....

Signature ....
Name ....
Position ....
Date ....

Staff in attendance

Midwife present...

Anaesthetist present...

Most senior obstetrician present, and status

....

Obstetrician called at ....hrs; arrived at ....hrs

Most likely cause

Uterine atony ☐

Trauma ☐

  Perineum intact ☐ Episiotomy ☐

  1st degree tear ☐ 2nd degree tear ☐

  3rd/4th degree tear ☐

  Episiotomy with extension ☐

Clotting disorder ☐

Retained products ☐

Placenta checked by ....

  Complete ☐ Ragged membranes ☐

  Retained products ☐

Oxytocics used

IV Syntocinon (40 units) started ☐ Time ....

2nd Syntometrine given ☐ Time given ....

Misoprostol 800 mcg given ☐ Time(s) given......

....

Bakri balloon in place? Yes ☐ No ☐

For woman who declines blood transfusion, use the local management pathway.

Further management

HDU chart ☐ Hourly MEWS ☐

Monitor pv loss ☐ IV fluids prescribed ☐

Obtain blood results and inform doctor ☐

Can Fragmin be given? Yes ☐ No ☐

At what time? .... or review at ....

Needs antibiotics? Yes ☐ No ☐ Prescribed ☐

Woman/ partner debriefed Yes ☐ No ☐

Time of next review ....

FIGURE 70.2 PPH documentation proforma.

Disseminated intravascular coagulopathy

71

Disseminated intravascular coagulopathy (DIC) should be anticipated in severe pre-eclampsia, APH, PPH, placental abruption, HELLP syndrome, acute fatty liver of pregnancy, amniotic fluid embolism and septicaemia.

Early involvement of the haematologist is vital.

71.1 INVESTIGATIONS

- FBC
- Group and cross-match 4–6 units of blood
- Obtain a coagulation profile

71.1.1 Features

- Low platelet count.
- Prolonged PT and APTT.
- Low fibrinogen (<2 g/L) and elevated FDP levels are indicative of decompensation.

Serial measurements of haemostatic indices are more informative than single readings.

71.2 TREATMENT

- High-dependency care
- Manage shock
- Liaise with the consultant haematologist (regarding blood product support)
- Treat the underlying cause – this is the cornerstone of management
- See the protocol for management of massive haemorrhage (Sections 66.6 and 66.7)
- Mechanical thromboprophylaxis

Delivery of the woman at known risk of haemorrhage

72

A higher risk of major bleeding at delivery should be anticipated in the following cases:

- Previous PPH
- Placenta praevia
- Significant uterine fibroids
- Previous myomectomy
- Placental abruption
- Multiple pregnancy
- APH
- Grandmultiparity
- Retained placenta
- Macrosomia
- Prolonged labour

If any of the prior applies:

- Insert a 14FG IV cannula during labour.
- FBC and group-and-save on admission.
- Empty the bladder in the third stage of labour.
- Active management of the third stage of labour.

A Syntocinon (oxytocin) infusion 40 units in 50 mL 0.9% saline (or Hartmann's) should be given for 4 hours after delivery.

72.1 IF SURGERY IS INDICATED

All elective and emergency surgery should be performed by a consultant or by an experienced obstetrician, with a consultant in attendance.

A senior anaesthetist should be involved.

Elective CS for placenta praevia and other potentially difficult cases should be scheduled for a session when a consultant anaesthetist is available.

- Consider interventional radiology.
- Consider cell salvage: alert perfusionist.
- Place two 14FG IV cannulas before surgery.

DOI: 10.1201/9781315099897-80

- Crossmatch 4 units of blood. These should be immediately available.
- Insert an arterial or CVP line (either preoperatively or when bleeding is excessive).

Liaise with the consultant haematologist in cases of coagulopathy.

See also management of PPH (Chapter 70) and management of major placenta praevia (Chapter 67).

Standards for administering blood transfusion

73

73.1 BACKGROUND

Despite improvements in the safety of blood transfusion, errors still occur, sometimes resulting in fatality. Each year between 2014 and 2021, more than 80% of reports submitted to SHOT (the UK agency responsible for promoting safety standards in blood transfusion) were related to transfusion errors, and most of these were preventable. The incidents arise from incorrect labelling of a blood sample, laboratory mistakes or administering the blood product to the wrong patient, and transfusion associated circulatory overload (TACO). Most of the errors occur not in emergency intraoperative situations but on the wards.

> There were 76 cases (of inappropriate and unnecessary transfusions) reported, with the largest group involving patients transfused on the basis of an erroneous laboratory value resulting from sampling, transcription or communication errors. A further significant category includes cases in which transfusion was given as a result of poor knowledge and decision making. There were two fatalities in this group: one from a massive over-transfusion, and one from under-transfusion, as well as one case of major morbidity. Attainment of appropriate knowledge and experience in transfusion medicine for clinical staff remains a major issue for medical educators.
>
> *Serious Hazards of Transfusion (SHOT) Annual Report, 2008*

> 'Errors continue to be the source of most SHOT reports (81.3%). While transfusions are largely safe, errors can result in patient harm. Many of these are caused by poor communication and distraction. These must be investigated using human factors principles-based incident investigations and appropriate mitigating measures implemented.'
>
> *SHOT Annual Report, 2021*

The single most important error resulting in mistransfusion is failure of the bedside checking procedure immediately before administering the transfusion.

This guidance is written to inform the training and practice of staff on the maternity unit, with a view to preventing errors in the administration of blood products. It should be read in conjunction with the hospital policy on blood transfusion.

Indications and techniques of blood transfusion are outside the scope of this chapter.

DOI: 10.1201/9781315099897-81

73.2 OBTAINING CONSENT

Except in emergencies or unconscious patients, the purpose, benefits and risks of blood transfusion should be explained to the woman. The alternatives to transfusion and the implications of declining a transfusion should also be discussed.

This discussion, and the woman's verbal consent to blood transfusion, should be documented. Encourage her to ask questions and provide her with written information.

73.3 COLLECTING A SPECIMEN FOR GROUP-AND-SAVE/CROSS-MATCH

See SHOT safety checklist – Safe-Transfusion-Practice-Transfusion-Checklist-July-2020.pdf (shotuk.org)

- The labels and cards must be completed *at the woman's bedside*, with the case notes available for reference.
- Do not use pre-labelled bottles. First obtain the blood specimen, and then label the bottles at the bedside.
- The blood specimen should not be obtained from an arm being used for infusion of IV fluids.
- When the doctor signs the request form, he or she is confirming that the sample is identified correctly.
- Previous transfusion records should be consulted.
- An IV cannula should be sited before the cross-matched blood is sent for.

73.4 CHECKING PROCEDURE FOR BLOOD TRANSFUSION

Ensure that *this* blood product is for *this* woman:

- Before transfusion, the labelling on the blood product must be checked against specific patient-identification details. This check must be carried out by two members of staff, one of whom must be a registered nurse or midwife.
- Read the wristband and check that this corresponds to the label on the blood product. Errors with wristbands may occur, so, if the woman is conscious, ask her to state her forename, family name and date of birth.
- If there are any discrepancies in spelling or identification number, transfusion should be withheld, and the blood transfusion department contacted immediately.
- Check the records of any previous blood grouping against the current report.
- There are two labels on the blood product bag, indicating:
  - Name of patient
  - Hospital number
  - Patient's blood group
  - Donor unit number

- ○ Compatibility type
- ○ Donor's blood group
- ○ Date and time of transfusion

These details must be checked against the form sent with the blood from the blood bank and signed. One label must be removed and put in the patient's records.

- The final bedside check provides an important opportunity to detect errors that may have been made earlier in the process of requesting blood.

! Patient identification errors and omissions continue to be of concern. In the [mistransfusions] reported, 6/40 (15.0%) events were caused by not properly identifying the patient. Patient misidentification in the transfusion laboratories have also been reported in 8 cases of [mistransfusion], all of these were mainly at the sample receipt and registration stage. In addition, there was one report where patient identification at testing was stated as the primary error. Accurate patient identification is fundamental to patient safety. One of the main SHOT recommendations in the 2019 Annual SHOT Report was that organisations must review all patient identification errors and establish the causes of patient misidentification. Recognising gaps in existing processes, use of electronic systems, empowerment of patients and staff will reduce these errors. Undertaking Positive Patient Identification (PPID) must be done at each step of the transfusion process when at the patient's bedside. This should be done using the ID band attached to the patient and wherever possible the patient should be included in the process. In emergency situations the patient's ID band, containing the core identifiers, must be used to confirm PPID prior to administering the transfusion. Not performing these checks at critical points such as pre-transfusion blood sampling or administration increases the risk of error which could result in the death of the patient. Blood is a 'living transplant' and should be treated with the same attentiveness as the transplant of a solid organ, administration of controlled drugs or provision of chemotherapy.

Serious Hazards of Transfusion (SHOT) Annual Report, 2021

73.5 DOCUMENTATION

The following should be entered in the case notes:

- Consent (verbal will suffice).
- Details of all blood products transfused (as noted earlier).
- The times at which transfusion commenced and ended.
- Observations, including pulse rate and temperature.
- Any transfusion reactions.

Errors should be documented and reported as prescribed in the hospital's policy on significant event reporting.

Observation should continue for 24 hours after blood transfusion.

Management of the woman who declines blood transfusion

74

Some women decline transfusion because of specific personal or religious beliefs. The main group of women who may refuse for religious reasons are members of the Jehovah's Witnesses.

If it is thought likely that a woman may refuse blood transfusion, then management of massive haemorrhage should be considered in advance.

74.1 ANTENATAL CARE

Discuss the risks of withholding blood transfusion (in a non-confrontational, non-judgemental manner). The woman should be offered the opportunity to read and discuss the guidance given next.

She should be asked if she is willing to receive blood transfusion in a life-threatening emergency, and her reply should be noted. This reply, given without duress, constitutes an advance decision. She should sign the appropriate form indicating her refusal of blood or blood products.

A copy of her advance decision document should be in her hospital records. It should be clear what interventions she will accept and which ones she does not want:

- ☐ Whole blood
- ☐ Red cells
- ☐ White cells
- ☐ Platelets
- ☐ FFP
- ☐ Blood products:
  - ☐ Albumin
  - ☐ Cryoprecipitate
  - ☐ Immunoglobulin
  - ☐ Coagulation factors
  - ☐ Autologous transfusion using blood salvage systems

- Check blood group and antibody status at booking, 30 weeks and 36 weeks.
- Arrange a consultation with the consultant obstetric anaesthetist.
- Check haemoglobin and serum ferritin at 36 weeks.
- Haematinics should be given throughout pregnancy to maximize iron stores.
- Discuss the management of peripartum bleeding, including the role of interventional radiology.

DOI: 10.1201/9781315099897-82

If an ultrasound scan shows a low-lying placenta, then the implications should be discussed with the woman.

> ! Blood storage for autotransfusion should not be suggested to pregnant women, since the amounts of blood required to treat massive obstetric haemorrhage are far more than the amount that could be donated during pregnancy.

The consultant obstetrician must be kept informed of any antenatal complications.

74.2 LABOUR

- On admission, inform the consultant obstetrician and consultant anaesthetist.
- Review the antenatal assessment as outlined earlier.
- Confirm with the woman what her wishes are.
- Note whether she is taking any drugs that could cause or aggravate bleeding.
- If a cell salvage device is to be used, alert the perfusionist.
- The third stage of labour should be managed actively.
- The woman should be observed closely for at least an hour after delivery.

If CS is necessary, it should be carried out by a consultant obstetrician if possible.

When the mother is discharged from hospital, she should be advised to report any bleeding promptly.

74.3 MANAGEMENT OF HAEMORRHAGE

The principle is to avoid delay. Rapid decision-making may be necessary, particularly regarding surgical intervention.

- Inform the consultant obstetrician.
- Inform the consultant anaesthetist.
- Inform the consultant haematologist.
- Promptly commence standard management (short of blood transfusion) of APH and PPH (Chapters 66 and 70).

The threshold for intervention should be lower than in other patients.

Extra vigilance should be exercised to quantify any abnormal bleeding and to detect complications, such as clotting abnormalities, as promptly as possible.

74.4 COMMUNICATION

- Keep the woman fully informed about what is happening. Information must be given in a professional way, ideally by someone whom the woman knows and trusts.

- Maintain a professional attitude. Do not lose the trust of the patient or her partner, since further decisions (e.g. regarding hysterectomy) may have to be made.
- If standard treatment is not controlling the bleeding, advise the woman that blood transfusion is strongly recommended. She is entitled to change her mind about a previously agreed treatment plan.
- Be satisfied that the woman is not being subjected to pressure from others. It is reasonable to ask the accompanying persons to leave the room for a while so that the doctor (with a midwife or other colleague) can ask the woman whether she is making her decision of her own free will.
- If the woman maintains her refusal to accept blood or blood products, then her wishes must be respected.

74.5 DRUGS AND INFUSIONS

Dextran should be avoided for fluid replacement because of its possible effects on haemostasis. IV crystalloid and plasma substitutes (Haemaccel or Gelofusine) should be used. In cases of severe bleeding, tranexamic acid and IV vitamin K should be given to the woman. Other drugs that have been recommended include desmopressin and methylprednisolone.

The advice of the haematologist should be sought before considering the use of heparin to combat DIC.

If the woman survives the acute episode and is transferred to ITU, management there should include erythropoietin, parenteral iron therapy and adequate protein for haemoglobin synthesis.

74.6 HYSTERECTOMY

Hysterectomy is usually a treatment of last resort in obstetric haemorrhage, but for a woman who declines blood transfusion any delay may increase the risk of death. The timing of hysterectomy is an on-the-spot decision for the consultant.

When hysterectomy is performed, the uterine arteries should be clamped as early as possible in the procedure. Subtotal hysterectomy can be just as effective as total hysterectomy and is quicker and safer.

In some cases, there may be a place for ligation of the internal iliac artery.

! If, despite all care, the woman dies, then her relatives require support like any other bereaved family.

74.7 MANAGEMENT OF STAFF

It is distressing for staff to have to watch a woman bleed to death or near death while refusing effective treatment. Support should be available for staff in these circumstances.

SECTION 4

Infection

Prophylactic antibiotics

75

75.1 CAESAREAN SECTION

WHO recommendation (2021): 'For antibiotic prophylaxis for caesarean section, a single dose of first-generation cephalosporin or penicillin should be used in preference to other classes of antibiotics.'

All women of normal BMI undergoing elective or emergency CS should have a single-dose prophylactic antibiotic: IV cefuroxime 750 mg or IV cefazolin 1 g given 30–60 minutes prior to skin incision (rather than intraoperatively after umbilical cord clamping).

If not possible (e.g. emergency surgery), administer as soon as possible after the incision.

If there are two or more of the following risk factors for postoperative wound infection, then consider giving a second dose or a full course of antibiotics:

- Prolonged rupture of membranes (>12 hours).
- Prolonged labour (>8 hours).
- Multiple vaginal examinations (>5 in the past 24 hours).
- Obesity (body mass index >30 kg/m2 at booking).

A second intraoperative dose should be given if blood loss is up to 1500 mL.

Due to the increased risk of necrotizing enterocolitis among preterm babies exposed to amoxicillin plus clavulanate (Augmentin), the use of amoxicillin plus clavulanate for antibiotic prophylaxis should be avoided before cord clamping for caesarean section of preterm infants.

75.2 CARDIAC DISEASE (SEE CHAPTER 49)

All women in labour and with a structural heart defect, prosthetic valve or history of endocarditis must have prophylactic antibiotics:

- CS: amoxicillin 1 g IV and gentamicin 120 mg IV (over 3 minutes), administered 30–60 min prior to procedure, then amoxicillin 500 mg 6 hours later. (Gentamicin dose: 3–4 mg/kg pre-pregnant weight.)
- Vaginal delivery: amoxicillin 1 g IV and gentamicin 120 mg IV (over 3 minutes) at onset of labour or ruptured membranes, then amoxicillin 500 mg 6 hours later.
- Woman allergic to penicillin or who has had more than a single dose of penicillin in the previous month: vancomycin 1 g by slow IV infusion (over at least 60 minutes) before delivery, then gentamicin 120 mg IV at induction of anaesthesia or at rupture of membranes.

DOI: 10.1201/9781315099897-84

75.3 GROUP B STREPTOCOCCI (GBS)

See Chapter 77.

75.4 PROLONGED RUPTURE OF FETAL MEMBRANES

Commence prophylactic antibiotics after 18 hours. Follow the same regimen as for GBS (Chapter 77). See also antibiotic use in PROM (Sections 37.2 to 37.5).

Intrapartum sepsis

76

Clinical features (not always present): pyrexia, hypothermia, hypotension, tachycardia, tachypnoea, hypoxia, impaired consciousness, diarrhoea, vomiting, cough, rash, urinary symptoms, oliguria.

Intrapartum pyrexia: Until proven otherwise, assume that the woman has sepsis. Inadequate treatment of intraoperative pyrexia can lead to escalation of sepsis and substantial maternal morbidity.

Implementation of the Sepsis Six within the first hour of diagnosing sepsis is associated with a 50% reduction in mortality.

Sepsis Six: Blood culture; Serum lactate; Urine output; Oxygen therapy; Intravenous antibiotics; Intravenous fluids.

76.1 PRINCIPLES

- Look for a focus of infection: respiratory, cardiac, urinary tract or other.
- Treat empirically with antibiotics while awaiting test results. Seek the advice of a microbiologist at an early stage regarding appropriate antibiotic therapy.
- For beta-haemolytic *Streptococcus pyogenes* (Lancefield Group A), the most appropriate antibiotic is a combination of Tazocin (piperacillin and the betalactamase inhibitor tazobactam) and an aminoglycoside.
- Beware of VTE presenting as pyrexia.
- Watch for fetal tachycardia.

76.2 ACTION PLAN

- FBC
- U/E
- CRP
- Send specimen for culture:
  - Vaginal swab
  - Endocervical swab
  - Midstream urine
  - Blood
  - Sputum and/or throat swab if respiratory symptoms present
- Serial serum lactate. Serum lactate level >2 mmol/L is a marker for septic shock
- Intravenous fluids
- IV antibiotics: co-amoxiclav 1.2 g every 8 hours or cefuroxime 1.5 g + metronidazole 500 mg every 8 hours will suffice as first-line therapy in women who are pyrexial but otherwise well

DOI: 10.1201/9781315099897-85

- In severe cases, add gentamicin or consider Tazocin (discuss with the microbiologist)
- Administer O_2, with a saturation target of 94%
- CTG
- Record temperature hourly
- Monitor urine output
- Inform the paediatrician
- Watch for deterioration to severe sepsis or septic shock
- Post-delivery, send the following for culture:
  - Swabs from baby
  - Placental swab

Hepatitis B and C

77

In the intrapartum care of a woman infected with hepatitis B or C virus (HBV or HCV), the aim is to reduce the chances of transmitting infection to the baby and/or staff. The risk of neonatal infection is variable.

Elective CS is not routinely indicated for HBV or HCV but may be offered to women co-infected with HCV and HIV.

Mother-to-child transmission of HBV can be reduced by giving the baby passive (immunoglobulin) and active (vaccination) immunization.

77.1 ACTION PLAN

- Admit into a designated room.
- Check the case notes for any instructions from the virologist regarding management.
- Universal precautions apply – wear disposable apron, gown, gloves, mask and spectacles.
- For CS and repair of episiotomy/perineal tear, consider the use of blunt needles.
- Obtain cord blood for hepatitis B surface antigen (HBsAg) and E core antibody (HBeAb).
- Disinfect boots, bed and other material with antiseptic.
- Alert the paediatric staff that the baby will need postexposure prophylaxis – within 12 hours of birth – see doses in the next section. Confirm that an immunization schedule is in place.

! • Do not use an FSE.
  • Do not perform FBS.

77.2 IMMUNIZATION

- Hepatitis B immunoglobulin: 200 IU IM, single dose, given within 24 hours of birth.
- Hepatitis B vaccine: 10 mg IM, within 24 hours of birth and at 1, 2 and 12 months.
- These injections should be given at separate sites.

77.3 BREASTFEEDING

It is safe for a mother with hepatitis B or hepatitis C to breastfeed her baby immediately after birth. As there is no vaccination against hepatitis C for the baby, breastfeeding should be temporarily stopped if the women's nipples or areola is cracked or bleeding.

Intrapartum antibiotic prophylaxis for group B streptococci

78

78.1 PRINCIPLES

From 1% to 2% of babies born to women who carry group B streptococci (GBS) will develop clinical infection. Although this transmission rate is low, the fatality rate in affected babies is high (15%–50%). Preterm infants have a ten times greater risk of acquiring GBS than do full-term infants.

Intrapartum antibiotic prophylaxis prevents vertical transmission and early-onset neonatal GBS.

Note: A GBS colony count $\geq 10^5$ CFU/mL warrants both acute treatment (at the time of diagnosis) and intrapartum antibiotic prophylaxis.

Asymptomatic GBS bacteriuria with colony count $<10^5$ CFU/mL does not require acute treatment but is an indication for intrapartum antibiotic prophylaxis.

78.2 RISK FACTORS

- Labour at <37 weeks' gestation.
- Prolonged rupture of membranes (>18 hours).
- Intrapartum pyrexia (>38°C, 100.4°F).
- Previous delivery of an infant with GBS.
- GBS urinary tract infection.
- Previous HVS showing GBS.
- Previous baby with neonatal GBS infection.

78.3 INDICATIONS FOR INTRAPARTUM GBS PROPHYLAXIS

- Previous neonate with GBS disease.
- GBS bacteriuria in this pregnancy.
- Positive GBS culture at ≥36 weeks, unless CS is performed with intact fetal membranes.
- Unknown GBS status and labour at <37 weeks or rupture of membranes >18 hours or intrapartum pyrexia.

DOI: 10.1201/9781315099897-87

78.4 INTRAPARTUM GBS PROPHYLAXIS NOT INDICATED

- CS performed before rupture of membranes, regardless of GBS status.
- Negative recto-vaginal GBS culture at ≥36 weeks.
- GBS colonization in a previous pregnancy but known to be negative in this pregnancy.

78.5 ACTION PLAN

For all women falling in the at-risk groups listed earlier:

- Send a low vaginal swab for culture.
- Check for allergy to penicillin.
- Give benzylpenicillin (penicillin G) 3 g IV load as soon as possible after onset of labour, then give 1.5 g every 4 hours until delivery. **If the woman is allergic to penicillin, give clindamycin 900 mg IV every 8 hours until she has delivered**.

For a woman with a high-risk penicillin allergy and whose GBS isolate is not sensitive to clindamycin, give intravenous vancomycin 20 mg/kg intravenously every 8 hours, with a maximum of 2 g per single dose. Monitor U/E.

- For intrapartum pyrexia, use a broad-spectrum antibiotic that covers GBS.
- If GBS is confirmed, flag the notes (a GBS sticker may be used).
- If GBS is confirmed, ensure that the woman is informed fully. Emphasize the need for prophylactic antibiotics.

Intrapartum antibiotic prophylaxis is not required for women undergoing CS in the absence of labour and with intact membranes.

- Membrane sweeping is not contraindicated.
- Water birth is not contraindicated.
- For rupture of membranes at ≥34 weeks, proceed with induction of labour. If <34 weeks, discuss the risks of prematurity versus risk of neonatal infection.

78.6 NEONATE

Observe for the following features of sepsis:

- Irritability
- Floppiness
- Skin discolouration
- Feeding problem

- Abnormal temperature
- Tachypnoea

Monitor vital signs at 0, 1 and 2 hours, and then every 2 hour until 12 hours.
The baby should be managed as outlined in Figure 78.1.

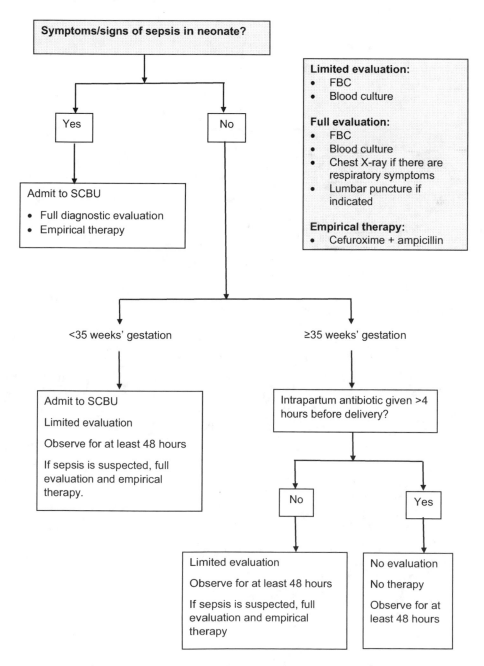

FIGURE 78.1   Management of a neonate whose mother received intrapartum antibiotic prophylaxis for GBS.

78.7 USEFUL CONTACT FOR PATIENTS

Group B Strep Support
PO Box 203
Haywards Heath
West Sussex RH16 1GF
UK
Tel: 01444 416176
www.gbss.org.uk

78.8 HELPLINE

0330 120 0796 (UK)

Genital herpes

79

About 90% of cases of genital herpes are caused by herpes simplex virus (HSV) type 2. It may present as painful vesicles or shallow ulcers, but there may be asymptomatic cervical lesions.

It may be a new (primary) infection or a recurrence. The risk of transmission to the baby is higher with primary infection (about 40%) than with recurrent infection (about 3%).

If labour commences <6 weeks after a first episode of genital herpes, there is insufficient time for the baby to be protected by maternal antibodies (HSV seroconversion), so the risk of transmission to the baby during vaginal birth is high.

If a primary infection is present at term or in labour, then elective CS should be offered; this reduces the risk of transmitting the infection to the baby.

For a woman with a vesicular lesion or a history of genital herpes:

- Examine the vulva and cervix.
- Obtain a cervical swab (and a vulval swab if lesions present) for viral culture if the diagnosis is unknown.
- If active herpes is present and fetal membranes are intact (or have just ruptured), offer CS.
- For primary (first episode) infection, this is the recommended mode of delivery.
- For recurrent infection, the risk to the baby is small (0%–3%) and must be weighed against the risk to the mother of a CS.
- If more than 4 hours have elapsed since membranes ruptured, ascending infection is likely to have occurred and CS is unlikely to reduce the risk of neonatal infection.
- Alert the paediatricians.
- Consult the genito-urinary physicians.
- Avoid invasive procedures such as amniotomy, FSE and FBS.
- Note that the use of aciclovir in pregnancy is off-label.

! It may be difficult to distinguish clinically between primary and recurrent genital herpes. If in doubt, treat as primary.

The decision pathway shown in Figure 79.1 is recommended.

Manage the neonate as advised by the paediatrician. Breastfeeding is not contraindicated unless there are herpetic breast lesions.

If the woman has a history of genital herpes and is HIV antibody positive, offer daily suppressive aciclovir 400 mg three times daily from 32 weeks of gestation to reduce the risk of transmission of HIV infection, especially if the plan is for a vaginal birth.

DOI: 10.1201/9781315099897-88

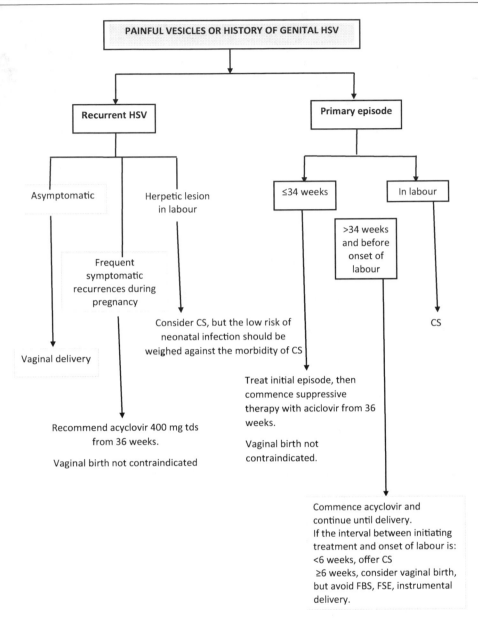

FIGURE 79.1   Decision pathway for mode of delivery in a woman with genital herpes.

Human immunodeficiency virus

80

To reduce the risk of mother-to-child transmission of human immunodeficiency virus (HIV), the woman should be on combined antiretroviral therapy (cART) during labour and breastfeeding. In women who have been treated appropriately with antiretroviral drugs, <10% of babies become infected with HIV.

The following events increase the risk of vertical transmission of HIV:

- Vaginal delivery
- Rupture of membranes >4 hours before delivery
- Preterm delivery (particularly <34 weeks)
- Use of FSE
- FBS
- Chorioamnionitis
- Breastfeeding
- High maternal viral load

80.1 MODE OF DELIVERY

Elective CS (usually at 38 weeks) with intact membranes reduces the risk of vertical transmission by at least 50%. However, if the mother has been on cART and viral load is undetectable, then vaginal delivery will carry about the same risk of vertical transmission as elective CS.

Regional analgesia is not contraindicated.

External cephalic version is not contraindicated if viral load is <50 HIV RNA copies/mL.

Water birth is not contraindicated if viral load is <50 HIV RNA copies/mL.

Vaginal birth after CS (VBAC) can be offered to women with a viral load <50 HIV RNA copies/mL.

Optimal mode of delivery determined by plasma viral load at 36 weeks:

- <50 HIV RNA copies/mL $\longrightarrow$ vaginal birth
- ≥400 HIV RNA copies/mL $\longrightarrow$ planned caesarean section at 38–39 weeks
- 50–399 HIV RNA copies/mL $\longrightarrow$ discuss balance of risks with the woman and virologist
- Regardless of the prior recommendations, the woman's wishes regarding mode of delivery should be respected

80.2 MANAGEMENT OF VAGINAL DELIVERY

- Alert the paediatrician.
- Treat any intercurrent infection.
- If the woman is on antiretroviral therapy, continue until delivery.
- If her viral load is <50 HIV RNA copies/mL, manage essentially as any other delivery. Intrapartum zidovudine infusion is not required.
- If her viral load is ≥50 HIV RNA copies/mL or viral count is not known.

Start zidovudine when in established labour or rupture of membranes is confirmed, or 3 hours before a scheduled CS.

The initial dose is 2 mg/kg IV over 1 hour (use the woman's weight at booking), and this is followed by 1 mg/kg/h until the cord is clamped. To prepare the required dilution:

- Remove 100 mL from a 500 mL bag of 5% glucose, leaving 400 mL.
- Take five vials each containing 20 mL of zidovudine at 10 mg/mL, and add this to the 400 mL of 5% glucose. This gives a solution of 1000 mg zidovudine in 500 mL, i.e. a concentration of 2 mg/mL. This may be kept for 24 hours if necessary.
- With this concentration, if the woman's weight is x (kg) then the *loading infusion rate* will be x (mL/h) and the *maintenance infusion rate* will be $0.5x$ (mL/h).
- If the woman is not on (or has only recently started) zidovudine, recommend nevirapine 200 mg orally immediately at onset of labour, and start IV zidovudine (see the aforementioned regime).
- Cleanse the vagina with chlorhexidine. Use Hibitane cream instead of KY Jelly.
- Avoid ARM, if possible.
- Expedite delivery if there is inadequate uterine activity after spontaneous rupture of membranes.
- The active phase of the second stage of labour should not exceed 1 hour.

80.3 OTHER MEASURES TO REDUCE THE RISK OF VERTICAL TRANSMISSION

- The use of FSE and FBS is contraindicated if viral load is ≥50 HIV RNA copies/mL or viral count not known.
- Avoid episiotomy, if possible.
- If instrumental delivery is required, forceps preferable to ventouse.
- Clamp the cord as quickly as possible after delivery.
- Suction the baby's mouth (**not trachea**) and nose immediately after delivery.
- Wash the baby immediately after birth in a warm bath.
- Administer antiretroviral medication to the baby as prescribed (liaise with the paediatricians).

80.4 AFTER DELIVERY

- Arrange a follow-up appointment in clinic
- Maintain confidentiality
- Neonatal care as directed by paediatrician

80.5 BREASTFEEDING

High-income countries: UK and US guidelines recommend avoidance of breastfeeding. However, if the mother opts to breastfeed, then respect her decision and support her.

Low-income countries: On the basis that ART is effective at preventing HIV transmission through breastfeeding as long as the mother is adherent to therapy, the WHO recommends that mothers living with HIV who are on ART and adherent to therapy should breastfeed exclusively for the first 6 months, and then add complementary feeding until 12 months of age.

80.6 PREPARATION FOR CAESAREAN SECTION

- Start zidovudine infusion 3–4 hours before operation. The initial dose is 2 mg/kg IV over 1 hour, followed by 1 mg/kg/h until the cord is clamped.
- Universal infection control measures apply.
- Use blunt needles.
- Use staples for skin.

80.7 PRELABOUR RUPTURE OF MEMBRANES AT TERM (PROM)

Induce labour immediately if viral load is well suppressed; otherwise offer CS. Aim for delivery within 24 hours of SROM. Ideally, the interval between rupture of membranes and delivery should be less than 4 hours.

80.8 PRETERM PRELABOUR RUPTURE OF MEMBRANES

If gestational age ≥34 weeks, manage as for PROM (previous section). May also need GBS prophylaxis.

If gestational age <34 weeks, assessment will have to be made as to the risk of HIV transmission compared with the risk of premature delivery. This assessment should involve obstetric, paediatric and infectious diseases staff.

There is no known contraindication to the use of steroids to promote fetal lung maturity in women with HIV.

80.9 CORD BLOOD

Cord blood should be taken for ultrasensitive HIV polymerase chain reaction (PCR), preferably in two EDTA bottles (one EDTA bottle will suffice if a sample sufficient to fill two bottles cannot be obtained). A clinical virology form must be completed, and 'ultrasensitive HIV PCR' should be written on the form.

To minimize needlestick injuries, a segment of cord should be steadied using two pairs of forceps.

80.10 CARE OF THE BABY

- Skin-to-skin contact should be established as soon as possible, unless declined by the mother.
- Bathe the baby.
- Administer vitamin K promptly, unless consent has been withheld.
- Administer antiretroviral therapy: nevirapine 2 mg/kg orally, one dose only, within 72 hours of birth (the sooner the better), and zidovudine 2 mg/kg every 6 hours orally, starting within 6 hours of birth and continued for 6 weeks.
- If the baby is premature or unable to tolerate oral medication, liaise with the HIV physician for IV medication.

80.11 INFECTION CONTROL

- Any needlestick injury should be managed as stipulated in the hospital policy.
- Standard personal protection equipment should be worn when undertaking any invasive procedures.

! Apply the 'Biohazard' policy and label to blood specimens and medical waste.

The woman with COVID-19

81

Most pregnant women with COVID-19 are either asymptomatic or have only mild or moderate symptoms. Of pregnant women admitted with symptomatic COVID-19:

- 1 of every 3 will require oxygen or other help to breathe.
- 1 in every 10 will be admitted to an intensive care unit.
- 1 in 5 of the will give birth to a preterm baby.

81.1 ACTION PLAN

- Inform multidisciplinary team:
  - Consultant obstetrician
  - Consultant anaesthetist
  - Consultant paediatrician/neonatologist
  - Midwife coordinator
  - Operating theatre coordinator
  - Infection control staff
- Implement infection control protocols for COVID-19 positive patients
- Manage in isolation room.
  - Provide surgical mask for woman and partner.
  - Ask if partner had any symptoms suggestive of COVID-19 in the preceding 10 days or had a fever within the last 48 hours.
  - One birth partner only.
  - PPE for staff.
  - Placenta must not be removed from the hospital.

81.2 CLINICAL CARE

- Assess the severity of COVID-19 symptoms.
- Monitor temperature, respiratory rate and oxygen saturation:
  - Hourly oxygen saturation monitoring.
  - Aim for oxygen saturation above 94%.
- Use continuous CTG monitoring for all women with symptomatic COVID-19 and any obstetric indication.

DOI: 10.1201/9781315099897-90

Mode of delivery is determined by obstetric and general medical status, not merely by the COVID-19 positive result.

Entonox® (50% nitrous oxide and 50% oxygen) can be safely offered with a standard single-patient microbiological filter.

Corticosteroids – if oxygen dependent give for a total of 10 days:

a. Oral prednisolone 40mg OD; or
b. IV hydrocortisone 80mg BD; or
c. Consider IV methyl prednisolone if severely unwell or needing ICU

If steroids used for fetal lung maturation use Dexamethasone 12mg IM 24 hourly (two doses) followed by either (a), (b) or (c) above for 10 days.

- Check anti-spike (anti-S) SARS-CoV-2 antibodies.
- Fetal scalp electrode monitoring and fetal blood sampling not contraindicated.
- Delayed cord clamping and skin-to-skin contact not contraindicated.
- Avoid general anaesthesia where possible as intubation may increase the risk of COVID-19 infection.

81.2.1 Water birth

- Water immersion/birth not contraindicated if she has asymptomatic COVID-19 infection or is SARS-CoV-2 swab negative.
- If she is symptomatic, with a cough, fever or feel unwell, water birth is contraindicated.
- Staff must wear waterproof PPE.

81.2.2 Thromboembolism prophylaxis

If on low-flow oxygen and at low risk of bleeding, offer a therapeutic dose of LMWH, unless birth is expected within 24 hours.

If on high-flow oxygen, CPAP, non-invasive ventilation or invasive ventilation, offer a prophylactic dose of LMWH.

Thromboprophylaxis for 10 days following hospital discharge.

Other obstetric emergencies

Paravaginal haematoma and cervical tear

82

82.1 PARAVAGINAL HAEMATOMA

There is a potential space lateral to the vaginal wall. The levatores ani muscles divide this space into upper and lower compartments. At childbirth, there may be bleeding into one of these compartments – see Figure 82.1.

- *Features*: Pain, swelling, urinary retention. May manifest as shock, in the absence of significant external bleeding.
- *Diagnosis*: Clinically, on palpation of a fluctuant mass in the lower vagina (infra-levator haematoma) or upper vagina (supra-levator haematoma). Could also be made by ultrasound scan or MR scan or CT scan with contrast.
- *Approaches to treatment*: Transvaginal surgical drainage; Laparotomy and drainage (supra-levator haematoma); Arterial embolization; Conservative management.

82.1.1 Action plan

- FBC
- Group-and-save
- Vital signs, EWS
- If in shock, manage as outlined on Sections 66.6 and 66.7
- Examine in theatre under general anaesthesia or epidural analgesia
- At examination under anaesthesia, ensure adequate exposure, with good lighting and an assistant
- Incision, drainage, ligation of bleeding vessels, application of a haemostatic agent, and packing of the infra-levator space, as may be required
- Ensure complete evacuation of the haematoma. A large incision may be required
- **After evacuation and repair, a tight pack should be inserted in the vagina. Specify when this should be removed**
- Give IV antibiotic: co-amoxiclav or cefuroxime/metronidazole
- Blood transfusion as required (there is a tendency to underestimate blood loss in a haematoma)

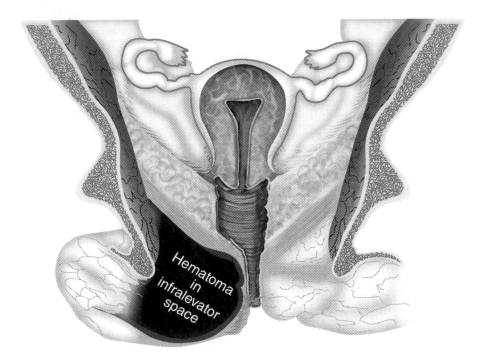

FIGURE 82.1   Paravaginal haematoma in the right lower levator compartment.

82.1.2 Conservative management

This should be considered if:

- She is haemodynamically stable.
- The haematoma is supra-levator (more difficult to evacuate transvaginally).

82.2 CERVICAL TEAR

Suspect this if there is postpartum haemorrhage despite the uterus being well-contracted and there is no evidence of vaginal or perineal tear.

Confirm by examination under anaesthesia in the operating theatre and with good lighting.

- Examine under anaesthesia. Inspect the cervix clockwise by serial clamping with sponge-holding forceps.
- The apex of the tear must be identified and repaired. If the apex cannot be seen, then a laparotomy is indicated.

A tear that is not bleeding can be allowed to heal spontaneously, without repair.

Rupture of the uterus

83

Early diagnosis depends on a high index of suspicion.
Suspect a ruptured uterus if there is:

- Sudden sharp abdominal pain followed by cessation of uterine contractions
- Abdominal tenderness
- Fetal distress (usually bradycardia)
- Vaginal bleeding
- Recession of the baby's head into the birth canal
- Maternal collapse
- Haematuria

! Any of the aforementioned in the presence of a uterine scar is strongly suggestive of uterine rupture.

83.1 ACTION PLAN

- Call the senior obstetrician and anaesthetist.
- Maintain the airway with oxygen via a facemask.
- Assess pulse and BP.
- Obtain IV access (14G or larger).
- FBC and clotting screen, and cross-match 6 units.
- Give IV Hartmann's solution and blood transfusion as necessary.
- Give CPR if necessary.
- Set up continuous CTG (apply a scalp electrode).
- Obtain consent for laparotomy, and possible hysterectomy, under general anaesthetic. The extent of the operation will depend on the extent of rupture, the amount of bleeding and the patient's future reproductive intentions.
- Give IV co-amoxiclav or cefuroxime/metronidazole.

83.2 PREVENTIVE CARE

In contemporary practice, most women who suffer a ruptured uterus have had a previous CS or an oxytocic drug, or both. All women undergoing a trial of vaginal delivery after CS should be informed of the risk of scar rupture (approximately 1 in 100).

DOI: 10.1201/9781315099897-93

In the presence of a uterine scar, a prostaglandin or Syntocinon (oxytocin) infusion should be used only with the prior approval of a consultant obstetrician, and the woman must be informed of the threefold increase in the risk of scar rupture.

Induction of labour in women with a previous CS should be in accordance with the protocol shown in Figure 35.3.

Vaginal birth after a previous CS should be managed as outlined in Chapter 34.

With Syntocinon induction or augmentation of labour, there should be continuous electronic fetal monitoring, and as much attention should be paid to the tocograph as to the cardiograph.

Shoulder dystocia

84

84.1 RISK FACTORS

- Large baby
- Diabetes
- Obesity (maternal BMI >30)
- Previous shoulder dystocia
- Secondary arrest after 8 cm cervical dilatation
- Prolonged first or second stage of labour
- Instrumental delivery

!
- 50% of shoulder dystocia occurs in normal-sized babies.
- More than 90% of macrosomic babies do not have dystocia.

84.2 RISKS TO MOTHER AND BABY

- Birth asphyxia
- Fractures
- Brachial plexus injury
- Perineal trauma

84.3 WHEN SHOULDER DYSTOCIA IS ANTICIPATED

- Discuss with the woman.
- Give epidural analgesia early in labour.
- Deliver in the lithotomy position.
- After delivery of the head, wait for the next uterine contraction before touching the baby. In most cases, the baby will be delivered spontaneously, with minimal accoucheur involvement. Many cases of shoulder dystocia are attributable to premature efforts to complete the delivery once the head has emerged from the birth canal.
- The registrar should be present at delivery.

DOI: 10.1201/9781315099897-94

84.4 TURTLE SIGN

The key to avoiding obstetric brachial plexus injury is to recognize, and respond appropriately to, the turtle sign. This is when the baby's head retracts against the mother's perineum (as a result of the baby's anterior shoulder impacting against the maternal pubic bone) – similar to a turtle pulling its head back into its shell. The baby's cheeks bulge out, its chin presses tightly on the perineum (you may find that you have to push back the perineum in order to deliver the chin), and the neck is not seen.

Once this sign appears, there should be no traction on the baby's head until the following action plan has been executed. When traction is subsequently applied, it should be axial, with no lateral flexion of the neck.

84.5 ACTION PLAN: 'HELPERR'

- **Help**: Call for help: senior obstetrician, second midwife, paediatrician and anaesthetist. A glance at the clock as you call for help or start manoeuvres is helpful. Nominate someone to record the timing and sequence of events. The woman's buttocks should be at the edge of the bed and her back should be flat on the bed. Do not panic!
- **Evaluate** for **episiotomy**.
- **Legs**: Place the legs in McRoberts position, with full flexion and abduction of the hips – the thighs should touch the abdomen. This manoeuvre requires two assistants. Attempt delivery in this position for 60 seconds. If this fails, the woman should remain in this position while the next manoeuvre is performed.
- **Pressure**: Apply suprapubic pressure (to the anterior shoulder), directed sideways, towards the anterior surface of the fetal chest. Pressure should be applied continuously or by a rocking motion. Traction should be applied on the baby's head and neck, without lateral flexion of the neck.

If the prior measures fail to deliver the shoulder (about 1 in 10 cases):

- **Enter** manoeuvres: start with the first of the following three manoeuvres and move to the next if unsuccessful in 60 seconds:
  - Insert the index and middle fingers behind the anterior shoulder and push it towards the baby's chest.
  - Woods' screw manoeuvre: apply pressure with two fingers behind the anterior shoulder and two fingers in front of the posterior shoulder.
  - Reverse Woods' screw: apply pressure with fingers behind the posterior shoulder.
- **Remove** the posterior arm. Deliver the posterior arm by following the humerus up to the elbow and flexing it. Grasp the wrist and sweep the arm across the chest until it is delivered.
- **Roll** the woman on to her hands and knees. Deliver the posterior arm by downward traction.
- If the previous drill is not successful and the baby is still alive, try either of the following:
  - Replace the baby's head and proceed to CS. To push back the head, first convert it to the occipitoanterior position. Also, do this with the aid of a tocolytic.
  - Perform a symphysiotomy.
- If the baby is dead, a cleidotomy may be performed.

84.6 AFTER DELIVERY

- Repair any perineal tear/episiotomy.
- Watch for PPH.
- Assess the baby to exclude brachial plexus injury or other injury.
- Review the events with the woman and her partner.
- Complete an incident form.

84.7 DOCUMENTATION

A local proforma is useful in capturing essential information. The following should be documented:

- The time of delivery of the head.
- The direction the head was facing after restitution.
- Which shoulder was the anterior shoulder.
- The manoeuvre(s) performed, including time and sequence.
- The time of delivery of the body.
- The staff in attendance and the time they arrived.
- Who else was present at delivery.
- The condition of the baby.
- Any deficit in motion of the extremities and which extremity(ies).
- Umbilical cord blood analysis.
- Any maternal injuries/complications.

All babies with actual or suspected brachial plexus injury, whether or not there was recorded shoulder dystocia, should be examined by the neonatologist on duty once the diagnosis is made or suspected.

Cord prolapse

85

Complete cord prolapse is when the umbilical cord slips below the presenting part, with ruptured membranes. In 'compound cord prolapse' (also known as 'occult cord prolapse'), the cord is alongside the presenting part, not below it.

Cord prolapse should always be excluded when spontaneous rupture of the membranes occurs and when amniotomy is performed.

The diagnosis may be suggested by sudden abnormalities on the CTG.

85.1 RISK FACTORS

- Breech presentation
- High head at onset of labour
- Multiple pregnancy
- Polyhydramnios
- Preterm labour

85.2 ACTION PLAN

- Ring the emergency bell.
- Summon the registrar, anaesthetist and anaesthetic practitioner, and paediatrician.
- Place the woman in the knee/chest (all-fours) position. If an epidural is sited, place her in the left lateral position.
- Push the presenting part above and away from the cord. Feel for pulsation but avoid unnecessary handling. Maintain this push while the woman is transferred to the operating theatre.

If cord pulsation is not palpable, use CTG and/or a scan to ascertain the status of the fetus.

- If cord pulsating, move the woman to the operating theatre immediately.
- Explain to the woman and her partner what is happening.
- Deliver by CS unless:
  - The cervix is fully dilated and the presenting part is below the ischial spines (in which case use ventouse or forceps delivery), or
  - The baby is not alive.
- Measure umbilical cord pH.
- After delivery, discuss the event with the woman and her partner.
- Documentation: provide a chronological account of events and management.

DOI: 10.1201/9781315099897-95

If for any reason delivery is delayed, fill the bladder with 500–750 mL 0.9% saline. This relieves cord compression directly as well as indirectly (by inhibiting uterine contractions) – but do not forget to empty the bladder before proceeding with CS.

If necessary, consider the use of terbutaline 250 mcg sc for tocolysis.

Anaphylaxis

86

A serious generalized or systemic hypersensitivity reaction of rapid onset. Could be life-threatening if emergency treatment is not given. May be induced by a drug, food or insect. Intramuscular adrenaline is first-line management.

86.1 PRESENTATION

- Itching
- Flushing
- Rash
- Nausea
- Vomiting
- Breathlessness
- Wheezing
- Oedema
- Tachycardia
- Hypotension
- Respiratory or cardiac collapse

86.2 WORLD ALLERGY ORGANIZATION CRITERIA FOR DIAGNOSIS OF ANAPHYLAXIS

Anaphylaxis is highly likely when any one of the following two criteria are fulfilled:

1. Acute onset of an illness with simultaneous involvement of the skin, mucosal tissue, or both. And at least one of the following:
   a. Respiratory compromise
   b. Reduced BP or associated symptoms of end-organ dysfunction (e.g. collapse, syncope, incontinence)
   c. Severe gastrointestinal symptoms, especially after exposure to non-food allergens.
2. Acute onset of hypotension or bronchospasm or laryngeal involvement after exposure to a known or highly probable allergen for that patient (minutes to several hours), even in the absence of typical skin involvement.

Differential diagnoses include acute asthma, anxiety attack, generalized urticaria, septic shock, pulmonary embolism.

DOI: 10.1201/9781315099897-96

86.3 ACTION PLAN

- Summon help
- Discontinue/remove the offending agent
- Assess airways, breathing and circulation, and commence basic life support if appropriate
- Position her appropriately:
  - Semi-recumbent position on the left side
  - Raise the feet to help restore BP
  - Place in a sitting position if in respiratory distress
  - Recovery position if unconscious
- Administer high flow oxygen 100%
- Give 0.5 mg adrenaline IM (i.e. 0.5 mL of 1: 1000 injection). Repeat every 10 minutes until BP and pulse are normal or help arrives
- Monitor vital signs and O_2 saturation
- Insert a 14FG or 16 FG IV cannula
- Give an IV infusion of Gelofusine or Haemaccel
- Check arterial blood gases
- For bronchospasm, give aminophylline 250 mg IV over 20 minutes
- Give chlorphenamine 10 mg IV, by slow infusion
- Consider giving hydrocortisone 100 mg IV
- Institute continuous electronic fetal monitoring if the woman is prenatal

Inverted uterus

87

Uterine inversion is when the *fundus* prolapses into the body of the uterus and beyond, to the cervix (Grade 1), the vagina (Grade 2), or the introitus (Grade 3). It may occur spontaneously or because of mismanagement of the third stage of labour. It causes severe pain and may result in shock without evidence of bleeding, due to vagal stimulation. Haemorrhagic shock can occur if inversion has followed, or is followed by, uterine atony.

Rapid colloid infusion may fail to improve the woman's condition, and care should be taken to avoid fluid overload.

87.1 ACTION PLAN

- If the woman is in shock, assess airways, breathing and circulation; summon help and commence basic life support if appropriate
- Exclude submucous fibroid (the uterus will be palpable abdominally)
- Maintain IV access (16–18G cannula) and give Hartmann's solution
- Facial oxygen
- FBC; Coagulation
- Cross-match 4 units of blood
- IV fluids
- Alert theatre team
- Reduce the inverted uterus
- Commence Syntocinon (oxytocin) infusion, 40 units in 500 mL 5% glucose following successful reduction

87.2 REDUCTION OF THE INVERSION

87.2.1 Manual reduction

- **If the inversion occurs during delivery**, it may be possible to replace the uterus immediately with Entonox or IM pethidine. If effective epidural analgesia is already in place, then this could be adequate. In all other circumstances, and **particularly if the woman is in shock**, reduction of an inverted uterus should be performed under a general anaesthetic.
- Consider relaxing the uterus with SC terbutaline.
- Reach the fundus of the uterus using the umbilical cord as a guide, and advance it into the abdominal cavity.

DOI: 10.1201/9781315099897-97

- **If the placenta has not separated**, replace the uterus and commence Syntocinon infusion (40 units in 500 mL Hartmann's solution), and then perform manual removal of the placenta. Do not attempt to remove the placenta before replacing the uterus.

87.3 HYDROSTATIC REDUCTION

- Exclude vaginal tear and rupture of the uterus before using this technique.
- Use *warm* saline (start with a 1 L bag) via a wide-bore giving set. The bag should be about 1 m above the patient (this gives a hydrostatic pressure of 100 cmH$_2$O), or use a pressure jacket. Do not use hypotonic fluid.
- The accoucheur covers the vaginal introitus with his/her hands, or with a 6 cm Silastic ventouse cup to provide a seal.
- **A general anaesthetic is not mandatory.**
- If the placenta has not separated, replace the uterus and commence Syntocinon infusion (40 units in 500 mL Hartmann's solution), and then perform manual removal of the placenta.
- Keep a record of the amounts of fluid infused into the vagina and released from it.

! Do not attempt to remove the placenta before replacing the uterus, since doing so could increase haemorrhage, shock and intravasation of fluid.

Rarely, it may be necessary to perform laparotomy and reduction from above.

Acute inversion may be complicated by pulmonary oedema from excessive IV fluids or, in cases of hydrostatic replacement, from fluid intravasation.

Discuss management of the third stage of labour in the next pregnancy.

Amniotic fluid embolism

88

This condition may occur suddenly in labour, at CS, or soon after delivery. The mortality rate is about 60%–80%. Morbidity in survivors is high. Cardiovascular collapse and respiratory symptoms are the most common initial presentations.

A high index of suspicion could be lifesaving. This rare condition must be suspected if there is:

- Disorientation/agitation/delirium
- Sudden shock (cardiovascular collapse)
- Chills
- Respiratory distress
- Cyanosis
- Fetal distress
- Coma
- Coagulopathy

If acute hypotension or cardiac arrest, acute hypoxia and coagulopathy occur during labour or CS or within 30 minutes postpartum and there is no other explanation (i.e. the differential diagnoses have been excluded), then a clinical diagnosis of amniotic fluid embolism can be made.

88.1 DIFFERENTIAL DIAGNOSES

- PE
- Myocardial infarction
- Mendelson's syndrome
- Cerebrovascular accident
- Total spinal
- Septic shock
- Substance abuse
- Placental abruption
- Eclampsia

88.2 MANAGEMENT

- Summon help
- Commence basic life support
- FBC

DOI: 10.1201/9781315099897-98

- Obtain a coagulation profile: PT, APTT and fibrinogen
- FDP/D-dimer
- U/E
- LFT
- Obtain IV access; give IV fluids
- Arterial line. Automated BP monitoring
- Central venous access
- Cross-match 4 units of blood
- Chest X-ray
- V/Q scan
- ECG
- Pulse oximetry
- Transthoracic or transesophageal echocardiography
- Insert a CVP line and arterial catheter
- Insert a urinary catheter
- CTG, if undelivered
- Inotropic support: epinephrine is the first-line agent
- Contact the consultant haematologist immediately – do not wait until coagulopathy is evident. Transfuse FFP, cryoprecipitate and platelets as advised by the haematologist
- Liaise with the consultant anaesthetist
- Give tranexamic acid
- Transfer to ITU as soon as possible. If the woman is undelivered, an urgent CS should be performed before transfer

Delivery should occur within 5 minutes of cardiac arrest if there is no response to initial resuscitation (neonatal outcome is dependent on a short cardiac arrest-to-delivery interval).

- Hysterectomy may be required if bleeding not controlled.
- Hydrocortisone is recommended.
- Other aspects of management are as outlined in Chapter 70 (management of massive haemorrhage).

Sudden maternal collapse

89

89.1 POSSIBLE CAUSES

- PPH (possibly concealed in broad ligament or paravaginal haematoma)
- Sepsis
- Pneumothorax
- PE
- Amniotic fluid embolism
- Cardiac arrhythmia
- Inverted uterus
- Myocardial infarction
- Left ventricular failure
- Hypoglycaemia
- Diabetic ketoacidosis
- Cerebrovascular accident
- Drug reaction
- Anaphylaxis
- Thyroid crisis
- Uterine rupture
- Peripartum cardiomyopathy
- Ruptured aneurysm

89.2 MANAGEMENT

- Assess airways, breathing and circulation.
- Crash call and commence basic life support if appropriate; otherwise, turn the woman to the left lateral position.
- If CPR is required, ensure that pressure on the inferior vena cava by the pregnant uterus is relieved by means of a wedge under the woman's side.
- Examine for signs of vaginal bleeding, peritonitis and breathing difficulties.
- Consider intubation (by the anaesthetist, with cricoid pressure by the assistant), to reduce the risk of pulmonary aspiration.
- Give oxygen using bag and mask, 6 L/min.
- Give an IV infusion of Haemaccel or Gelofusine.
- If the woman is in pain, give IM pethidine 50–100 mg immediately.

DOI: 10.1201/9781315099897-99

89.3 INVESTIGATIONS

- FBC
- U/E
- LFT
- Coagulation screen
- Blood gases
- Group and cross-match
- Arterial line
- ECG
- Urinary catheter
- Portable chest X-ray

If the woman is diabetic, check her blood sugar with a glucometer and if indicated give an infusion of 50 mL 50% glucose. Inform the on-call medical registrar.

If resuscitation has been unsuccessful after 5 minutes, proceed to CS – not only to save the baby but also to increase the mother's chances of survival.

Latex allergy

90

For the treatment of anaphylaxis, see Chapter 86.

90.1 RISK FACTORS

- History of multiple surgical procedures
- History of atopy (hay fever, asthma, dermatitis or food allergy)
- Previous anaphylactic episode of unknown cause, particularly if associated with surgery or dental treatment
- Occupational exposure to latex

A latex-free pack for emergency use should always be available on the delivery suite.

90.2 CARE OF THE WOMAN ALLERGIC TO LATEX

- Case notes, patient identification band and room door should carry warnings of latex allergy.
- Labour should be conducted in a latex-free room.

All surfaces, including the bed frame, should be wiped clean.

- Latex free gloves only.
- Prepare a trolley with latex-free gloves, catheters, surgical tape, IV equipment and tourniquets for possible emergency use.
- Inform the anaesthetist.
- Management of IV drugs:
  - Draw up in latex-free syringes.
  - Do not reconstitute or inject through rubber bungs.
- Beware of latex BP cuffs.
- Prepare a back-up theatre (to be latex-free) in case an emergency CS is required. The minimum dust-settling time is 2 hours.
- Drugs used to treat allergic reactions should be ready for use.

The following should not be used or left exposed in the care of a woman who is allergic to latex:

- Latex gloves
- Foley catheter

DOI: 10.1201/9781315099897-100

- Entonox rubber tubing
- Elasticated straps for CTG monitor
- Rubber tourniquet
- Sphygmomanometer tubing
- Elastoplast
- Rubber mattress covers on theatre tables
- Other rubber products

90.3 OPERATING THEATRE (ELECTIVE OR EMERGENCY PROCEDURE)

If possible, she should be first on the list.

- Only essential personnel should be in theatre.
- Put up notices on theatre doors, marking the theatre as a latex-free room, and keep the doors shut.
- Removal of all latex items from theatre, anaesthetic room, scrub room, postop recovery room.

SECTION 6

Stillbirths and congenital abnormalities

Checklist for fetal loss at 13–23 weeks

91

91.1 PARENTS

- The parents should be given the opportunity to see and hold the fetus.
- Has a minister of religion been requested?
- The parents should be offered a photograph.
- The parents should be informed about the choice of hospital or private funeral. An information leaflet should be provided.
- Post-mortem examination should be discussed:
  - Has consent been given?
  - Has consent *not* been given?
- An appropriate bereavement pack should be provided.
- Has anti-D been given, if required?
- A follow-up appointment should be made.
- The woman should be seen by a doctor before discharge home.

91.2 COMMUNICATION

- Arrange suppression of mail for parent education classes, antenatal clinic and other antenatal activities.
- The antenatal clinic should be informed of the fetal loss.
- The GP should be informed by telephone/fax and letter.

91.3 FORMS/ADMINISTRATION

- Complete all forms per local protocol.
- Complete the fetal loss register.
- Arrangements should be made for transport to the mortuary.
- Comply with local policy on sensitive disposal of fetal tissue.

Intrauterine fetal demise

92

The care received during and after stillbirth may have lasting impact on the parents' wellbeing. It can help reduce the chances that the parent(s) will progress from a physiological to a pathological grief process.

The key elements in the management of a woman and her partner after a perinatal loss are communication; emotional support; support in decision-making, particularly in relation to holding the baby and post-mortem examination; and investigations to determine the cause of perinatal loss.

92.1 PRINCIPLES

- Be sure of the diagnosis before informing the woman.
- Keep the woman and her partner fully informed of what is happening.
- Show a caring attitude, but also give the woman and her partner the time and space that they require.
- As much as possible continuity of carer should be maintained, so that a relationship of empathy and trust is sustained and the parent is protected from distress associated with repetition of the same questions and answers.
- The investigations performed will depend on whether there was an obvious cause of fetal loss.
- The issue of consent for post-mortem examination is probably best brought up when discussing the cause of death.

92.2 DIAGNOSIS (IF NOT MADE BEFORE ADMISSION)

The first indication might be absence of fetal movement or inability to pick up fetal heart tones.

The obstetrician should perform an ultrasound scan. If fetal heart pulsation is not seen, the diagnosis should be confirmed by a practitioner who holds a formal qualification in ultrasound scanning. Inform the woman that fetal heart pulsation has not been seen but that a further scan is required and will be performed as soon as possible. Inform the consultant.

The senior obstetrician should discuss diagnosis and management with the woman. Decisions must be made regarding when and how to deliver the baby.

Administer mifepristone 200 mg orally, under supervision.

The GP, community midwife and health visitor should be informed, and antenatal appointments cancelled.

DOI: 10.1201/9781315099897-103

92.3 ACTION PLAN

Ideally, mifepristone should have been administered 36–48 hours before admission.

- Admit into a designated room.
- Discuss tests, including post-mortem examination of the baby. Document which tests the woman/couple have consented to.
- Provide information booklets on funeral arrangements and post-mortem examination.
- Ensure compliance with national policies and legislation; see Human Tissue Authority. Code A: Guiding principles and the fundamental principle of consent. HTA; May 2020. Code A (hta.gov.uk)
- Document consent for tests. In the UK, use a consent form that complies with the Human Tissue Act 2004, Human Tissue (Scotland) Act 2006 and the HTA's codes of practice. These laws require that specific consent should be obtained for each of the following: post-mortem examination, genetic testing, retention of organs, retention of DNA, imaging and use of materials for education or research.

A standard form for 'Consent to a hospital post mortem examination on a baby or child' is available.

- Induction of labour: see later.
- Investigations: see later.
- Consider antibiotic treatment.
- Discuss funeral arrangements – private or hospital burial – or disposal by the pathology laboratory.
- Offer counselling and provide details of support groups.
- If possible, avoid artificial rupture of membranes (risk of infection).
- Ask the parents if they wish to name the baby. Record the name in the notes.
- Examine the baby: wash, weigh, measure and label; check for abnormalities.
- Dress the baby (after examination, always keep the baby clothed).
- Parents should be allowed to see or hold the baby for as long as they wish.
- A photograph should be taken of the baby.
- A stillbirth certificate should be completed and signed.
- Ascertain the parent(s)' wishes: some parents may want the midwife or doctor to remain in the room and support them for a while after the demise of their baby while others will want a period of privacy.
- Prescribe medication to suppress lactation:
  - Cabergoline 1 mg orally, single dose.
  - Bromocriptine 2.5 mg twice daily for 14 days is a less expensive option but carries more risks; it should not be given to women with hypertension, coronary artery disease or any mental disorder.
- Arrange a follow-up appointment.

92.4 INVESTIGATIONS

92.4.1 Mother

92.4.1.1 Maternal blood tests

- FBC
- HbA1c (glycated haemoglobin)
- Blood group antibodies

- Thyroid function tests
- Bile salts
- Kleihauer test
- Lupus anticoagulant
- Anticardiolipin antibodies
- Coagulation screen
- TORCH screen (universal bottle, virology card): *Toxoplasma*, rubella, cytomegalovirus and hepatitis antibodies
- Parvovirus B19 screen
- Chromosome analysis, if not known
- Any other clinically indicated blood test

92.4.1.2 Urine

- Perform a drugs screen on a urine sample, if there is a suspicion of drug misuse.

92.4.1.3 Vaginal swab

- Take a vaginal swab (during routine examination before inducing labour) for microscopy and culture.

92.4.1.4 Placenta

- Swab for culture
- Send to pathology (for histology tests) in a bucket with formalin and a histology card

92.4.2 Fetus

- Take a full-depth fetal skin biopsy (0.5 cm^3) from the axilla for cytogenetics/FISH
- Do not clean the skin before biopsy
- Skin biopsy culture usually fails in macerated stillbirth
- Take a cord or cardiac blood sample (at least 0.5 mL into a 1–2 mL lithium heparin paediatric tube) for FBC, chromosome analysis and culture
- Take swabs from nose, throat, ear and umbilicus for culture
- Take photographs
- Take an X-ray of the fetus
- A post-mortem should be offered (see preceding Action plan)

92.5 INDUCTION OF LABOUR

Ensure that the fetal lie is longitudinal before induction of labour. If the lie is abnormal then the senior obstetrician should discuss version with the woman.

If fetal demise has occurred in mid-trimester, follow the algorithm described in Chapter 93.

If demise has occurred in the third trimester, assess the cervix and proceed as follows:

- **Cervix favourable**: perform amniotomy and commence a Syntocinon (oxytocin) infusion.
- **Cervix unfavourable for amniotomy but cervical score >5**: insert prostaglandin E_2 (PGE_2, dinoprostone) gel 1 mg. Repeat 4 hours later if the cervix remains unfavourable for amniotomy.

- **Cervical score <5, and no contraindications to gemeprost**: insert a gemeprost 1 mg pessary; repeat every 3 hours until labour is induced or amniotomy is feasible.
- **Cervical score <5 and gemeprost contraindicated**: use dinoprostone gel 2 mg. If required, a further dose of dinoprostone gel 1 mg may be given 4 hours later.

> ! Gemeprost should not be used in grandmultiparous women or in women with uterine scar.

If the cervix remains unfavourable for amniotomy despite two doses of dinoprostone gel, consider using extra-amniotic prostaglandin (see later).

If labour is not induced after five doses of gemeprost, allow 12–24 hours and then commence extra-amniotic prostaglandin as follows:

- One ampoule containing 5 mg of dinoprostone should be dissolved in 0.5 mL ethanol and 50 mL 0.9% saline. This gives a 100 µg/mL solution.
- Obtain a 12–14FG Foley catheter with a 30 mL balloon. Fill the dead space with 3 mL of the solution you have prepared.
- Under aseptic conditions, insert the catheter through the cervix and inflate the balloon.
- Start infusion at an initial rate of 1 mL/h, increasing to 2 mL/h if there is no uterine response after 4 hours.
- When the catheter falls out, amniotomy may be performed.

> ! Note that dinoprostone potentiates the effect of Syntocinon on the uterus.

If labour is not induced despite the measures described previously, further management will be determined by the consultant, based on the circumstances and preferences of the woman.

For twin delivery after 24 weeks when one twin is known to have died in utero before viability, the dead twin has to be registered as a stillbirth; it is assigned the gestational age of the live twin.

92.6 SUPPORT GROUP

Sands (Stillbirth & Neonatal Death Charity)
Sands, 10–18 Union Street, London, SE1 1SZ.
Helpline (UK): 0808 164 3332
email: helpline@sands.org.uk
Website: www.sands.org.uk/

Mid-trimester termination of pregnancy for fetal abnormality

93

The principles of management are as outlined for intrauterine fetal demise (Chapter 92). Ensure that the statutory forms for termination of pregnancy have been completed.

93.1 INVESTIGATIONS

These will depend on the nature of the abnormality.

93.2 PRENATAL DIAGNOSIS OF CHROMOSOMAL ABNORMALITY

- Take a full-depth fetal skin biopsy (0.5 cm^3) for cytogenetics/FISH.
- Take a sample of cord (2–3 cm in length) and a sample of placental membrane from around the cord-insertion site.
- Take a cord or cardiac blood sample (at least 0.5 mL into a 1–2 mL lithium heparin paediatric tube).

Send solid specimens in dry pots – **do not use formalin**. If transport has to be delayed overnight, store at 4°C; **do not freeze**. Ensure that containers are labelled properly.

93.3 ULTRASOUND SCAN DIAGNOSIS OF STRUCTURAL ABNORMALITY OR EXTERNAL APPEARANCE SUGGESTIVE OF ANEUPLOIDY

The procedure is the same as outlined previously.

DOI: 10.1201/9781315099897-104

93.4 SCAN DIAGNOSIS OF NEURAL TUBE DEFECT, WITH NO OTHER MALFORMATION OR RECURRENCES IN FAMILY

Cytogenetic diagnosis is not routinely required in these cases.

93.5 GENETIC EXAMINATION OF FETUSES AND SAMPLES

Only fetuses (and samples) aborted in the following circumstances should be sent to the laboratory:

- Prenatal diagnosis of chromosomal abnormality.
- Scan diagnosis of structural abnormality (in the case of neural tube defects, those with other abnormalities or where there has been recurrence in the family).
- Miscarriage where the baby has obvious malformations.

93.6 INDUCTION OF LABOUR

As part of the process of obtaining consent for this procedure, an information leaflet should be provided. The leaflet should include contact details.

93.6.1 Procedure

- The woman takes one tablet (200 mg) of mifepristone, witnessed by staff.
- She is observed for 1 hour. If vomiting occurs, give prochlorperazine 12.5 mg IM and repeat mifepristone.
- The woman is discharged home. The discharge information should include a contact telephone number.
- 36–48 hours later, the woman attends the ward and the procedure is explained again.
- Misoprostol 800 µg (or gemeprost 1 mg) is inserted into the posterior fornix.
- If the fetus/products have not been expelled, give oral misoprostol 400 µg every 4 hours (or gemeprost 1 mg pessary every 3 hours) up to a maximum of four doses.
- Analgesia should be given as required (co-codamol every 4 hours or diamorphine 5–10 mg IM every 4 hours).
- Record BP, pulse and temperature hourly.
- If the first course of treatment was successful and the woman is in a stable condition, discharge home, inform the GP, and confirm follow-up arrangements.
- If the first course of treatment was not successful, allow 12 hours from the last dose before commencing a second course of gemeprost pessaries, as mentioned previously.

93.7 CONTRAINDICATIONS

The use of mifepristone is contraindicated in the following cases:

- Allergy to mifepristone
- Chronic renal failure
- Long-term corticosteroid therapy
- Clotting disorders or anticoagulant therapy
- Anaemia ([Hb] <8.5 g/dL)
- Smoker aged ≥35 years
- Suspected ectopic pregnancy

The use of misoprostol or gemeprost is contraindicated in the following cases:

- Allergy to prostaglandins
- Severe asthma

93.8 CAUTION

Use mifepristone with caution in the following cases:

- Asthma
- Chronic obstructive airway disease
- Cardiovascular disease
- Renal failure
- Liver failure
- Prosthetic heart valves

Use misoprostol and gemeprost with caution in the following cases:

- Cerebrovascular disease
- Coronary artery disease
- Severe peripheral vascular disease, including hypertension

Further reading for Part III

Caesarean section

American College of Obstericians and Gynecologists Practice Bulletin No. 199. Use of prophylactic antibiotics in labor and delivery. *Obstet Gynecol.* 2018;132(3):e103–19. doi: 10.1097/AOG.0000000000002833

Anorlu RI, Maholwans B, Hofmeyr GJ. Methods of delivering the placenta at caesarean section. *Cochrane Database Syst Rev.* 2008;3:CD004737

Lucas DN, Yentis SM, Kinsella SM, et al. Urgency of caesarean section: A new classification. *J R Soc Med.* 2000;93:346–50

Nabhan AF, Allam NE, Hamed Abdel-Aziz Salama M. Routes of administration of antibiotic prophylaxis for preventing infection after caesarean section. *Cochrane Database Syst Rev.* 2016 Jun 17;2016(6):CD011876. doi: 10.1002/14651858.CD011876.pub2

National Institute for Health and Clinical Excellence. *Caesarean Birth: NICE Guideline.* NICE; 2021 Mar

Waterfall H, Grivell RM, Dodd JM. Techniques for assisting difficult delivery at caesarean section. *Cochrane Database Syst Rev.* 2016 Jan 31;2016(1):CD004944. doi: 10.1002/14651858.CD004944.pub3

Recovery of obstetric patients

The Royal College of Anaesthetists. Guidelines for the Provision of Anaesthetic Services (GPAS). *Chapter 9: Guidelines for the Provision of Anaesthesia Services for an Obstetric Population.* RCA, 2022 Mar

Warren J, Fromm RE Jr, Orr RA, Rotello LC, Horst HM, American College of Critical Care Medicine. Guidelines for the inter- and intrahospital transport of critically ill patients. *Crit Care Med.* 2004 Jan;32(1):256–62. doi: 10.1097/01.CCM.0000104917.39204.0A

High-dependency care

Royal College of Anaesthetists, Royal College of Obstetricians and Gynaecologists, Royal College of Midwives, Intensive Care Society. *Care of the Critically Ill Woman in Childbirth; Enhanced Maternal Care 2018.* London: RCA, 2018

Umar A, Ameh CA, Muriithi F, Mathai M. Early warning systems in obstetrics: A systematic literature review. *PLoS One.* 2019;14(5):e0217864. doi:10.1371/journal.pone.0217864

Failed intubation drill

Mushambi MC, Kinsella SM, Popat M, Swales H, Ramaswamy K, Winton AL, Quinn A. Obstetric anaesthetists' association and difficult airway society guidelines for the management of difficult and failed tracheal intubation in obstetrics*. *Anaesthesia.* 2015;70:1286–306

Patil S, Sinha P, Krishnan S. Successful delivery in a morbidly obese patient after failed intubation and regional technique. *Br J Anaesth.* 2007;919–20

Instrumental delivery

Edozien LC. Towards safe practice in instrumental delivery. *Best Prac Res Clin Obstet Gynaecol.* 2007;21:639–55

Murphy DJ, Strachan BK, Bahl R, On behalf of the Royal College of Obstetricians and Gynaecologists: Assisted vaginal birth. *BJOG.* 2020;127:e70–112

DOI: 10.1201/9781315099897-105

Verma GL, Spalding JJ, Wilkinson MD, Hofmeyr GJ, Vannevel V, O'Mahony F. Instruments for assisted vaginal birth. *Cochrane Database Syst Rev.* 2021;9. Art. No.: CD005455. DOI: 10.1002/14651858.CD005455.pub3

Trial of vaginal delivery after a previous caesarean section

The American College of Obstetricians and Gynaecologists. *Vaginal Birth After Cesarean Delivery.* Practice Bulletin No. 205, 2019 Feb

Edozien LC. Vaginal birth after Caesarean section: What information should women be given? *Clinical Risk.* 2007;13:127–30

Kabiri D, Masarwy R, Schachter-Safrai N, Masarwa R, Hirsh Raccah B, Ezra Y, Matok I. Trial of labor after cesarean delivery in twin gestations: Systematic review and meta-analysis. *Am J Obstet Gynecol.* 2019;220(4):336–47. doi: 10.1016/j.ajog.2018.11.125

Royal College of Obstetricians and Gynaecologists. *Birth After Previous Caesarean Birth.* Green-top Guideline No. 45, 2015 Oct

Visser GHA. Trial of vaginal breech delivery in carefully selected women is worth considering- Fruit for thought! *Eur J Obstet Gynecol Reprod Biol.* 2020;252:574–5. doi: 10.1016/j.ejogrb.2020.03.048

Induction of labour

Kehl S, Weiss C, Rath W. Balloon catheters for induction of labor at term after previous cesarean section: A systematic review. *Eur J Obstet Gynecol Reprod Biol.* 2016 Sep;204:44–50. doi: 10.1016/j.ejogrb.2016.07.505

The National Institute for Health and Care Excellence (NICE). *Inducing Labour.* NICE Guideline [NG207], 2021 Nov. Available at: www.nice.org.uk/guidance/indevelopment/gid-ng10082

Royal College of Midwifery. *Blue Top Guidance No. 2.* Midwifery Care for Induction of Labour. Available at: https://www.rcm.org.uk/media/3706/midwifery-care-for-induction-of-labour-information-for-women-and-families-a4-2019-12pp_1-002-003.pdf

Tsakiridis I, Mamopoulos A, Athanasiadis A, Dagklis T. Induction of labor: An overview of guidelines. *Obstet Gynecol Surv.* 2020;75(1):61–72. doi: 10.1097/OGX.0000000000000752. PMID: 31999354

Antenatal corticosteroid therapy

American College of Obstetricians and Gynaecologists. Prelabor rupture of membranes: ACOG practice bulletin, number 217. *Obstet Gynecol.* 2020;135(3):e80–97. doi: 10.1097/AOG.0000000000003700

Roberts D, Brown J, Medley N, Dalziel SR. Antenatal corticosteroids for accelerating fetal lung maturation for women at risk of preterm birth. *Cochrane Database Syst Rev.* 2017;3(3):CD004454. doi: 10.1002/14651858.CD004454.pub3

Royal College of Obstetricians and Gynaecologists. Care of women presenting with suspected preterm prelabour rupture of membranes from 24 + 0 weeks of gestation. Green-top guideline no. 73. *BJOG.* 2019;126: e152–66. doi:10.1111/1471-0528.15803

Stock SJ, Thomson AJ, Papworth S. The Royal College of Obstetricians and Gynaecologists: Antenatal corticosteroids to reduce neonatal morbidity and mortality. Green-top guideline No. 74. *BJOG* 2022;129

Preterm prelabour rupture of membranes

Kenyon S, Boulvain M, Neilson JP. Antibiotics for preterm rupture of membranes. *Cochrane Database Syst Rev.* 2013;12:CD001058. doi: 10.1002/14651858.CD001058.pub3

Preterm uterine contractions

Flenady V, Reinebrant HE, Liley HG, Tambimuttu EG, Papatsonis DN. Oxytocin receptor antagonists for inhibiting preterm labour. *Cochrane Database Syst Rev.* 2014;6:CD004452. doi: 10.1002/14651858.CD004452.pub3

National Institute of Health and Care Excellence. *Preterm labour and birth.* NICE Guideline [NG25]. Published 2015 Nov; Updated 2022 Jun

Papatsonis DN, van Geijn HP, Ader HJ, et al. Nifedipine and ritodrine in the management of preterm labour: A randomised multicentre trial. *Obstet Gynecol* 1997;90:230–4

Wilson A, Hodgetts-Morton VA, Marson EJ, Markland AD, Larkai E, Papadopoulou A, Coomarasamy A, Tobias A, Chou D, Oladapo OT, Price MJ, Morris K, Gallos ID. Tocolytics for delaying preterm birth: A network meta-analysis (0924). *Cochrane Database Syst Rev*. 2022 Aug 10;8(8):CD014978. doi: 10.1002/14651858. CD014978.pub2

Deliveries at the lower margin of viability

American Academy of Pediatrics Committee on Fetus and Newborn. American College of Obstetricians and Gynecologists Committee on Obstetric Practice. Perinatal care at the threshold of viability. *Pediatrics* 1995;96:974–6

Costeloe K, Hennessy E, Gibson AT, et al. The EPICure study: Outcomes to discharge from hospital for infants born at the threshold of viability. *Paediatrics* 2000;106:659–71

Lemyre B, Daboval T, Dunn S, Kekewich M, Jones G, Wang D, Mason-Ward M, Moore GP. Shared decision making for infants born at the threshold of viability: A prognosis-based guideline. *J Perinatol*. 2016 Jul;36(7):503–9. doi: 10.1038/jp.2016.81

Multiple pregnancy

Barrett JF. Twin delivery: Method, timing and conduct. *Best Pract Res Clin Obstet Gynaecol*. 2014;28(2):327–38. doi: 10.1016/j.bpobgyn.2013.12.008

Dufour PH, Vinatier S, Vanderstichele S, et al. Intravenous nitroglycerin for intrapartum podalic version of the second twin in transverse lie. *Obstet Gynecol*. 1998;92:416–19

National Collaborating Centre for Women's and Children's Health (UK). *Multiple Pregnancy: The Management of Twin and Triplet Pregnancies in the Antenatal Period*. London: RCOG Press;2011

Occipito-posterior position

Hunter S, Hofmeyr GJ, Kulier R. Hands and knees posture in late pregnancy or labour for fetal malposition (lateral or posterior). *Cochrane Database Syst Rev*. 2007;4:CD001063

Simkin P. The fetal occiput posterior position: state of the science and a new perspective. *Birth*. 2010;37(1):61–71. doi: 10.1111/j.1523-536X.2009.00380.x

Malpresentation

Pilliod RA, Caughey AB. Fetal malpresentation and malposition: Diagnosis and management. *Obstet Gynecol Clin North Am*. 2017;44(4):631–43. doi: 10.1016/j.ogc.2017.08.003

Talaulikar VS, Arulkumaran S. Malpositions and malpresentations of the fetal head. *Obstetrics, Gynaecology & Reproductive Medicine*. 2012;22(6):155–61

Breech presentation

American College of Obstetricians and Gynecologists. Mode of term singleton breech delivery. ACOG Committee Opinion No. 745. *Obstet Gynecol*. 2018;132:e60–3

Impey LWM, Murphy DJ, Griffiths M, Penna LK. On behalf of the Royal College of Obstetricians and Gynaecologists: Management of breech presentation. *BJOG*. 2017;124:e151–77

External cephalic version

Hofmeyr GJ, Kulier R, West HM. External cephalic version for breech presentation at term. *Cochrane Database Syst Rev*. 2015;2015(4):CD000083. doi: 10.1002/14651858.CD000083.pub3

Impey LWM, Murphy DJ, Griffiths M, Penna LK. On behalf of the Royal College of Obstetricians and Gynaecologists: External cephalic version and reducing the incidence of term breech presentation. *BJOG*. 2017;124:e178–92

Weill Y, Pollack RN. The efficacy and safety of external cephalic version after a previous caesarean delivery. *Aust N Z J Obstet Gynaecol*. 2017;57(3):323–6. doi: 10.1111/ajo.12527

The woman with genital mutilation

Larsen U, Okonofua FE. Female circumcision and obstetric complications. *Int J Gynaecol Obstet.* 2002;77:255–65

Royal College of Nursing. *Female Genital Mutilation: An RCN Resource for Nursing and Midwifery Practice.* Fourth edition. RCN, 2019

Royal College of Obstetricians and Gynaecologists. *Female Genital Mutilation and Its Management.* Green-top Guideline No. 53, 2015 Jul

The obese woman in labour

Denison FC, Aedla NR, Keag O, Hor K, Reynolds RM, Milne A, Diamond A, On behalf of the Royal College of Obstetricians and Gynaecologists: Care of women with obesity in pregnancy. Green-top guideline no. 72. *BJOG* 2018;72

Perineal tear

Fernando RJ, Sultan AH, Kettle C, Thakar R. Methods of repair for obstetric anal sphincter injury. *Cochrane Database Syst Rev.* 2013;12:CD002866. doi: 10.1002/14651858.CD002866.pub3

Kettle C, Dowswell T, Ismail KM. Absorbable suture materials for primary repair of episiotomy and second degree tears. *Cochrane Database Syst Rev.* 2010;10(6):CD000006. doi: 10.1002/14651858.CD000006.pub2

Kettle C, Dowswell T, Ismail KM. Continuous and interrupted suturing techniques for repair of episiotomy or second-degree tears. *Cochrane Database Syst Rev.* 2012;11(11):CD000947. doi: 10.1002/14651858.CD000947.pub3

Royal College of Obstetricians and Gynaecologists. *The Management of Third- and Fourth-Degree Perineal Tears.* Green-top Guideline No. 29. RCN, 2015 Jun

Heart disease in labour

Regitz-Zagrosek V, Roos-Hesselink JW, Bauersachs J, et al. 2018 ESC guidelines for the management of cardiovascular diseases during pregnancy. *Eur Heart J.* 2018;39(34):3165–241

Schaufelberger M. Cardiomyopathy and pregnancy. *Heart.* 2019;105(20):1543–51. doi: 10.1136/heartjnl-2018-313476

Peripartum cardiomyopathy

Cho SH, Leonard SA, Lyndon A, Main EK, Abrams B, Hameed AB, Carmichael SL. Pre-pregnancy obesity and the risk of peripartum cardiomyopathy. *Am J Perinatol.* 2021;38(12):1289–96. doi: 10.1055/s-0040-1712451

Cooney R, Scott JR, Mahowald M, Langen E, Sharma G, Kao DP, Davis MB. Heart rate as an early predictor of severe cardiomyopathy and increased mortality in peripartum cardiomyopathy. *Clin Cardiol.* 2022;45(2):205–13. doi: 10.1002/clc.23782

Mi-Jeong Kim, Mi-Seung Shin. Practical management of peripartum cardiomyopathy. *Korean J Intern Med.* 2017;32(3):393–403

Olagundoye VV, Seow Y, Ashworth MA. Peripartum cardiomyopathy: A forgotten diagnosis? *Hosp Med.* 2003;64:50–1

Pre-eclampsia

Brodie H, Malinow AM. Anaesthetic management of preeclampsia/eclampsia. *Int J Obstet Anesth.* 1999;8:110–24

Duley L, Gülmezoglu AM, Henderson-Smart DJ, Chou D. Magnesium sulphate and other anticonvulsants for women with pre-eclampsia. *Cochrane Database Syst Rev.* 2010;2010(11):CD000025. doi: 10.1002/14651858.CD000025.pub2

Idama TO, Lindlow SW. Magnesium sulphate: A review of clinical pharmacology applied to obstetrics. *BJOG* 1998;105:260–8

Sridharan K, Sequeira RP. Drugs for treating severe hypertension in pregnancy: A network meta-analysis and trial sequential analysis of randomized clinical trials. *Br J Clin Pharmacol.* 2018;84(9):1906–16. doi: 10.1111/bcp.13649

Stocks G. Preeclampsia: pathophysiology, old and new strategies for management. *Eur J Anaesthesiol.* 2014;31(4):183–9. doi: 10.1097/EJA.0000000000000044

Eclampsia

Cleary EM, Racchi NW, Patton KG, Kudrimoti M, Costantine MM, Rood KM. Trial of intrapartum extended-release nifedipine to prevent severe hypertension among pregnant individuals with preeclampsia with severe features. *Hypertension*. 2022 Oct 3. doi: 10.1161/HYPERTENSIONAHA.122.19751. Epub ahead of print

Duley L, Henderson-Smart DJ, Walker GJ, Chou D. Magnesium sulphate versus diazepam for eclampsia. *Cochrane Database Syst Rev*. 2010;2010(12):CD000127. doi: 10.1002/14651858.CD000127.pub2

Fishel Bartal M, Sibai BM. Eclampsia in the 21st century. *Am J Obstet Gynecol*. 2022;226(2S):S1237–53. doi: 10.1016/j.ajog.2020.09.037

Lam MTC, Dierking E. Intensive care unit issues in eclampsia and HELLP syndrome. *Int J Crit Illn Inj Sci*. 2017;7(3):136–41. doi: 10.4103/IJCIIS.IJCIIS_33_17

National Institute for Health and Clinical Excellence. *Hypertension in Pregnancy: Diagnosis and Management*. Clinical Guideline [CG107]. NICE, 2010 Aug

Diabetes mellitus

American College of Obstetricians and Gynecologists. ACOG practice bulletin no. 190: Gestational diabetes mellitus. *Obstet Gynecol*. 2018;131(2):e49–64. doi: 10.1097/AOG.0000000000002501

American College of Obstetricians and Gynecologists' Committee on Practice Bulletins – Obstetrics. ACOG practice bulletin no. 201: Pregestational diabetes mellitus. *Obstet Gynecol*. 2018;132(6):e228–48. doi: 10.1097/AOG.0000000000002960

Feig DS, Berger H, Donovan L. Diabetes and pregnancy. *Can J Diabetes*. 2018;42:255–82

Joint British Diabetes Societies for Inpatient Care. *Management of Glycaemic Control in Pregnant Women with Diabetes on Obstetric Wards and Delivery Units*. JBDS, 2017 May

Lamont T, Cousins D, Hillson R. Safer administration of insulin: Summary of a safety report from the national patient safety agency. *BMJ*. 2010;341:c5269

National Institute for Health and Care Excellence guideline. *Diabetes in Pregnancy: Management from Pre-Conception to the Postnatal Period*. 2015 Feb. Available at: www.nice.org.uk/guidance/ng3

Royal College of Midwives. *Caring for Pregnant Women with Pre-existing and Gestational Diabetes*. RCM, 2022 Sep

Yap Y, Modi A, Lucas N. The peripartum management of diabetes. *BJA Educ*. 2020;20(1):5–9. doi: 10.1016/j.bjae.2019.09.008

Asthma (acute exacerbation in labour)

National Asthma Education and Prevention Program. *Working Group Report on Managing Asthma During Pregnancy: Recommendations for Pharmacologic Treatment – Update 2004*. US Department of Health and Human Services. National Institutes of Health, National Heart, Lung, and Blood Institute. NIH Publication No. 05–5236, 2005 Mar

Popa M, Peltecu G, Gica N, Ciobanu AM, Botezatu R, Gica C, Steriade A, Panaitescu AM. Asthma in pregnancy: Review of current literature and recommendations. *Maedica (Bucur)*. 2021;16(1):80–7. doi: 10.26574/maedica.2020.16.1.80

Scottish Intercollegiate Guidelines Network and British Thoracic Society. *SIGN158 British Guideline on the Management of Asthma: A National Clinical Guideline*. Revised edition. SIGN158, 2019 Jul

Epilepsy

Bhatia M, Adcock JE, Mackillop L. The management of pregnant women with epilepsy: A multidisciplinary collaborative approach to care. *The Obstetrician and Gynaecologist* 2017;19(4): 279–88. doi:10.1111/tog.12413

Royal College of Obstetricians and Gynecologists. *Epilepsy in Pregnancy Green-top Guideline No. 68*. London: RCOG, 2016 Jun

Systemic lupus erythematosus

Buchanan NMM, Khamashta MA, Kerslake S, et al. Practical management of pregnancy in systemic lupus erythematosus. *Fet Mat Med Rev*. 1993;5:223–30

Castro-Gutierrez A, Young K, Bermas BL. Pregnancy and management in women with rheumatoid arthritis, systemic lupus erythematosus, and obstetric antiphospholipid syndrome. *Med Clin North Am*. 2021;105(2):341–53. doi: 10.1016/j.mcna.2020.10.002

Mascola MA, Repke JT. Obstetric management of the high-risk lupus pregnancy. *Rheum Dis Clin North Am*. 1997;23:119–32

Other connective tissue disorders

Erez Y, Ezra Y, Rojansky N. Ehlers-Danlos type IV in pregnancy: A case report and a literature review. *Fetal Diagn Ther*. 2008;23(1):7–9. doi: 10.1159/000109218

Goland S, Elkayam U. Pregnancy and marfan syndrome. *Ann Cardiothorac Surg*. 2017;6(6):642–53. doi: 10.21037/acs.2017.10.07

Williams A, Grantz K, Seeni I, Robledo C, Li S, Ouidir M, Nobles C, Mendola P. Obstetric and neonatal complications among women with autoimmune disease. *J Autoimmun*. 2019;103:102287. doi: 10.1016/j.jaut.2019.05.015

The rhesus-negative woman

Qureshi H, Massey E, Kirwan D, Davies T, Robson S, White J, Jones J, Allard S, British Society for Haematology. BCSH guideline for the use of anti-D immunoglobulin for the prevention of haemolytic disease of the fetus and newborn. *Transfus Med*. 2014 Feb;24(1):8–20. doi: 10.1111/tme.12091

Thromboembolism prophylaxis

Royal College of Obstetricians and Gynaecologists. *Reducing the Risk of Venous Thromboembolism During Pregnancy and the Puerperium*. Green-top Guideline No. 37a, 2015 Apr

Acute venous thromboembolism and pulmonary embolism

American College of Obstetricians and Gynecologists' Committee on Practice Bulletins – Obstetrics. ACOG Practice Bulletin No. 196: Thromboembolism in Pregnancy. *Obstet Gynecol*. 2018;132(1):e1–17. doi: 10.1097/AOG.0000000000002706

Dedionigi C, Le Gal G, Righini M. D-dimer to rule out venous thromboembolism during pregnancy: A systematic review and meta-analysis. *J Thromb Haemost*. 2021;19(10):2454–67. doi: 10.1111/jth.15432

Gutiérrez García I, Pérez Cañadas P, Martínez Uriarte J, García Izquierdo O, Angeles Jódar Pérez M, García de Guadiana Romualdo L. D-dimer during pregnancy: Establishing trimester-specific reference intervals. *Scand J Clin Lab Invest*. 2018;78(6):439–42. doi: 10.1080/00365513.2018.1488177

Royal College of Obstetricians and Gynaecologists. *Thromboembolic Disease in Pregnancy and the Puerperium: Acute Management*. Green-top Guideline No. 37b, 2015 Apr

Major haemoglobinopathy

Howard J, Oteng-Ntim E. The obstetric management of sickle cell disease. *Best Pract Res Clin Obstet Gynaecol*. 2012;26(1):25–36. doi: 10.1016/j.bpobgyn.2011.10.001

Romano D, Craig H, Katz D. Management of cesarean delivery in a parturient with sickle cell disease. *Int J Obstet Anesth*. 2020;41:104–7. doi: 10.1016/j.ijoa.2019.09.001

Royal College of Obstetricians and Gynaecologists. *Management of Sickle Cell Disease in Pregnancy*. Green-top Guideline No. 61, 2011 Jul

Inherited coagulation disorders: haemophilia and von Willebrand disease

Castaman G, James PD. Pregnancy and delivery in women with von Willebrand disease. *Eur J Haematol*. 2019;103(2):73–9. doi: 10.1111/ejh.13250

Chi C, Lee CA, Shiltagh N, Khan A, Pollard D, Kadir RA. Pregnancy in carriers of haemophilia. *Haemophilia*. 2008;14(1):56–64. doi: 10.1111/j.1365-2516.2007.01561.x

Davies J, Kadir R. The management of factor XI deficiency in pregnancy. *Semin Thromb Hemost*. 2016;42(7):732–40. doi: 10.1055/s-0036-1587685

Walker ID, Walker JJ, Colvin BT, et al. Investigation and management of haemorrhagic disorders in pregnancy: Haemostasis and thrombosis task force. *J Clin Pathol* 1994;47:100–8

Immune thrombocytopenic purpura

Eslick R, McLintock C. Managing ITP and thrombocytopenia in pregnancy. *Platelets*. 2020;31(3):300–6. doi: 10.1080/09537104.2019.1640870

Stavrou E, McCrae KR. Immune thrombocytopenia in pregnancy. *Hematol Oncol Clin North Am*. 2009;23(6):1299–316. doi: 10.1016/j.hoc.2009.08.005

Thrombophilia

American College of Obstetricians and Gynecologists' Committee on Practice Bulletins – Obstetrics. ACOG practice bulletin no. 197: Inherited thrombophilias in pregnancy. *Obstet Gynecol*. 2018;132(1):e18–34. doi: 10.1097/AOG.0000000000002703

Croles FN, Nasserinejad K, Duvekot JJ, Kruip MJ, Meijer K, Leebeek FW. Pregnancy, thrombophilia, and the risk of a first venous thrombosis: Systematic review and Bayesian meta-analysis. *BMJ*. 2017 Oct 26;359:j4452. doi: 10.1136/bmj.j4452

Gestational thrombocytopenia

American College of Obstetricians and Gynecologists. ACOG practice bulletin no. 207: Thrombocytopenia in pregnancy. *Obstet Gynecol*. 2019;133(3):e181–93. doi: 10.1097/AOG.0000000000003100

Fadiloglu E, Unal C, Tanacan A, Portakal O, Beksac MS. 5 years' experience of a tertiary center with thrombocytopenic pregnancies: Gestational thrombocytopenia, idiopathic thrombocytopenic purpura and hypertensive disorders of pregnancy. *Geburtshilfe Frauenheilkd*. 2020;80(1):76–83. doi: 10.1055/a-0865-4442

Major placenta praevia

Jain V, Bos H, Bujold E. Guideline no. 402: Diagnosis and management of placenta previa. *J Obstet Gynaecol Can*. 2020;42(7):906–17.e1. doi: 10.1016/j.jogc.2019.07.019

Jauniaux E, Alfirevic Z, Bhide AG, Belfort MA, Burton GJ, Collins SL, Dornan S, Jurkovic D, Kayem G, Kingdom J, Silver R, Sentilhes L, Royal College of Obstetricians and Gynaecologists. Placenta praevia and placenta accreta: Diagnosis and management. Green-top guideline no. 27a. *BJOG*. 2019;126(1):e1–48. doi: 10.1111/1471-0528.15306

Ruiter L, Kok N, Limpens J, Derks JB, de Graaf IM, Mol B, Pajkrt E. Incidence of and risk indicators for vasa praevia: A systematic review. *BJOG*. 2016 Jul;123(8):1278–87. doi: 10.1111/1471-0528.13829

Placenta accreta spectrum

American College of Obstetricians and Gynaecologists & Society for Maternal-Fetal Medicine. Obstetric consensus statement: Placenta accreta spectrum. *Obstetrics and Gynaecology* 2018;132:e259–75

Hobson SR, Kingdom JC, Murji A, et al. No. 383 – screening, diagnosis, and management of placenta accreta spectrum disorders. *J Obstet Gynaecol Can*. 2019;41:1035–49

Jauniaux ERM, Alfirevic Z, Bhide AG, Belfort MA, Burton GJ, Collins SL, Dornan S, Jurkovic D, Kayem G, Kingdom J, Silver R, Sentilhes L. On behalf of the Royal College of Obstetricians and Gynaecologists. Placenta praevia and placenta accreta: Diagnosis and management. Green-top guideline no. 27a. *BJOG*. 2018;27

Jauniaux ERM, Ayres-de-Campos D, Langhoff-Roos J, et al. FIGO placenta accreta diagnosis and management expert consensus panel. FIGO classification for the clinical diagnosis of placenta accreta spectrum disorders. *Int J Gynaecol Obstet*. 2019;146:20–4

Retained placenta

Cummings K, Doherty DA, Magann EF, Wendel PJ, Morrison JC. Timing of manual placenta removal to prevent postpartum hemorrhage: Is it time to act? *J Matern Fetal Neonatal Med*. 2016;29(24):3930–3. doi: 10.3109/14767058.2016.1154941

Franke D, Zepf J, Burkhardt T, Stein P, Zimmermann R, Haslinger C. Retained placenta and postpartum hemorrhage: Time is not everything. *Arch Gynecol Obstet*. 2021;304(4):903–11. doi: 10.1007/s00404-021-06027-5

Kumar N, Jahanfar S, Haas DM, Weeks AD. Umbilical vein injection for management of retained placenta. *Cochrane Database Syst Rev*. 2021;3(3):CD001337. doi: 10.1002/14651858.CD001337.pub3

Postpartum haemorrhage

Anorlu RI, Maholwana B, Hofmeyr GJ. Methods of delivering the placenta at caesarean section. *Cochrane Database Syst Rev*. 2008;3:CD004737

Guidelines for Intraoperative Cell Salvage. *Intraoperative Cell Salvage Education*. Available at: www.transfusion guidelines.org

Mavrides E, Allard S, Chandraharan E, Collins P, Green L, Hunt BJ, Riris S, Thomson AJ. On behalf of Royal College of Obstetricians and Gynaecologists: Prevention and management of postpartum haemorrhage. *BJOG*. 2016;124:e106–49

Price N, B-Lynch C. Technical description of the B-Lynch brace suture for treatment of massive postpartum hemorrhage and review of published cases. *Int J Fertil Womens Med*. 2005;50(4):148–63

Royal College of Obstetricians and Gynaecologists. *Blood Transfusion in Obstetrics*. Green-top Guideline No. 47; 2015 May

World Health Organization. *Updated WHO Recommendation on Tranexamic Acid for the Treatment of Postpartum Haemorrhage*. Geneva, Switzerland: World Health Organization, 2017. Available at: https://apps.who.int/iris/bitstream/handle/10665/259379/WHO-RHR-17.21-eng.pdf;sequence=1

Disseminated intravascular coagulopathy

Cunningham FG, Nelson DB. Disseminated intravascular coagulation syndromes in obstetrics. *Obstet Gynecol*. 2015;126(5):999–1011. doi: 10.1097/AOG.0000000000001110

Erez O, Othman M, Rabinovich A, Leron E, Gotsch F, Thachil J. DIC in pregnancy – pathophysiology, clinical characteristics, diagnostic scores, and treatments. *J Blood Med*. 2022;13:21–44. doi: 10.2147/JBM.S273047

Delivery of the woman at known risk of haemorrhage

Dahlke JD, Mendez-Figueroa H, Maggio L, Hauspurg AK, Sperling JD, Chauhan SP, Rouse DJ. Prevention and management of postpartum hemorrhage: A comparison of 4 national guidelines. *Am J Obstet Gynecol*. 2015;213(1):76.e1–10. doi: 10.1016/j.ajog.2015.02.023

Gonzalez-Brown V, Schneider P. Prevention of postpartum hemorrhage. *Semin Fetal Neonatal Med*. 2020;25(5):101129. doi: 10.1016/j.siny.2020.101129

Management of the woman who declines blood transfusion

Scharman CD, Burger D, Shatzel JJ, Kim E, DeLoughery TG. Treatment of individuals who cannot receive blood products for religious or other reasons. *Am J Hematol*. 2017;92(12):1370–81. doi: 10.1002/ajh.24889

Zeybek B, Childress AM, Kilic GS, Phelps JY, Pacheco LD, Carter MA, Borahay MA. Management of the Jehovah's witness in obstetrics and gynecology: A comprehensive medical, ethical, and legal approach. *Obstet Gynecol Surv*. 2016 Aug;71(8):488–500. doi: 10.1097/OGX.0000000000000343

Prophylactic antibiotics

Committee on Practice Bulletins-Obstetrics. ACOG practice bulletin no. 199: Use of prophylactic antibiotics in labor and delivery. *Obstet Gynecol*. 2018 Sep;132(3):e103–19. doi: 10.1097/AOG.0000000000002833

World Health Organization. *WHO Recommendation on Prophylactic Antibiotics for Women Undergoing Caesarean Section*. Geneva: World Health Organization; 2021. Licence: CC BY-NC-SA 3.0 IGO

Intrapartum sepsis

Annane D. Body temperature in sepsis: A hot topic. *Lancet* 2018;6(3):162–3. doi: 10.1016/S2213-2600(18)30003-1

Bowyer L, Robinson HL, Barrett H, Crozier TM, Giles M, Idel I, Lowe S, Lust K, Marnoch CA, Morton MR, Said J, Wong M, Makris A. SOMANZ guidelines for the investigation and management sepsis in pregnancy. *Aust N Z J Obstet Gynaecol.* 2017;57(5):540–51. doi: 10.1111/ajo.12646

Conde-Agudelo A, Romero R, Jung EJ, Garcia Sánchez ÁJ. Management of clinical chorioamnionitis: an evidence-based approach. *Am J Obstet Gynecol.* 2020;223(6):848–69. doi: 10.1016/j.ajog.2020.09.044

Royal College of Obstetricians and Gynaecologists, *Bacterial Sepsis in Pregnancy.* Green – top Guideline No. 64a, 2012 Apr

Shields A, de Assis V, Halscott T. Top 10 Pearls for the recognition, evaluation, and management of maternal sepsis. Obstet Gynecol. 2021;138(2):289–304. doi: 10.1097/AOG.0000000000004471

Intrapartum antibiotic prophylaxis for group B streptococci

American College of Obstetricians and Gynecologists. *Prevention of Group B Streptococcal Early-Onset Disease in Newborns.* Committee Opinion No. 797, 2020 Feb

NHS Resolution. *Case Story Group B Streptococcus (GBS) in Pregnancy and Early Onset Infection in the Neonate.* NHS, 2021 Jun

Ohlsson A, Shah VS. Intrapartum antibiotics for known maternal group B streptococcal colonization. *Cochrane Database Syst Rev.* 2014 Jun 10;6:CD007467. doi: 10.1002/14651858.CD007467.pub4

Royal College of Obstetricians and Gynaecologists. Prevention of early-onset neonatal group B streptococcal disease. Green-top guideline no. 36. *BJOG.* 2017;124(12):e280–305. doi: 10.1111/1471-0528.14821

Genital herpes

American College of Obstetricians and Gynecologists. Management of genital herpes in pregnancy: ACOG practice bulletin number 220. *Obstet Gynecol.* 2020;135(5):e193–202. doi: 10.1097/AOG.0000000000003840

British Association for Sexual Health and HIV (BASHH) and the Royal College of Obstetricians and Gynaecologists (RCOG). *Management of Genital Herpes in Pregnancy.* Consensus Guideline, 2014 Oct

Money DM, Steben M. No. 208-guidelines for the management of herpes simplex virus in pregnancy. *J Obstet Gynaecol Can.* 2017;39(8):e199–205. doi: 10.1016/j.jogc.2017.04.016

Sénat MV, Anselem O, Picone O, Renesme L, Sananès N, Vauloup-Fellous C, Sellier Y, Laplace JP, Sentilhes L. Prevention and management of genital herpes simplex infection during pregnancy and delivery: Guidelines from the French College of Gynecologists and Obstetricians (CNGOF). *Eur J Obstet Gynecol Reprod Biol.* 2018;224:93–101. doi: 10.1016/j.ejogrb.2018.03.011

Human immunodeficiency virus

American College of Obstetricians and Gynaecologists. *Labor and Delivery Management of Women with Human Immunodeficiency Virus Infection.* Committee Opinion Number 751. ACOG, 2018 Sep

British HIV Association. *British HIV Association Guidelines for the Management of HIV in Pregnancy and Postpartum 2018 (2020 Third Interim Update).* British HIV Association Guidelines for the Management of HIV in Pregnancy and Postpartum 2018 (2020 third interim update). Available at: www.bhiva.org

Chilaka VN, Konje JC. Human immunodeficiency virus infection in pregnancy. *Eur J Obstet Gynecol Reprod Biol.* 2021;256:484–91. doi: 10.1016/j.ejogrb.2020.11.034

Harris K, Yudin MH. HIV Infection in pregnant women: A 2020 update. *Prenat Diagn.* 2020;40(13):1715–21. doi: 10.1002/pd.5769

World Health Organization, United Nations Children's Fund. *Guideline: Updates on HIV and Infant Feeding: The Duration of Breastfeeding, and Support from Health Services to Improve Feeding Practices Among Mothers Living with HIV.* Geneva: World Health Organization, 2016

COVID-19 infection in labour

Royal College of Obstetricians and Gynaecologists & Royal College of Midwives. *Coronavirus (COVID-19) Infection in Pregnancy. Information for Healthcare Professionals.* Version 15. Published 2022 Mar 7

Cervical tear and paravaginal haematoma

Bellussi F, Cataneo I, Dodaro MG, Youssef A, Salsi G, Pilu G. The use of ultrasound in the evaluation of postpartum paravaginal hematomas. *Am J Obstet Gynecol MFM.* 2019;1(1):82–8. doi: 10.1016/j.ajogmf.2019.03.002

Stobie W, Krishnan D. Large concealed paravaginal haematoma: A case report of an occult postpartum haemorrhage. *Case Rep Womens Health.* 2021;30:e00311. doi: 10.1016/j.crwh.2021.e00311

Rupture of the uterus

Elagwany AS, Fawzy A. Silent uterine rupture associated with the use of misoprostolduring second trimester pregnancy termination in primigravid. *Arch J Perinat Med.* 2015;21(1):57–9

Jayaprakash S, Muralidhar L, Sampathkumar G, Sexsena R. Rupture of bicornuate uterus. *BMJ Case Rep.* 2011;2011:bcr0820114633. doi: 10.1136/bcr.08.2011.4633

Shoulder dystocia

American College of Obstetricians and Gynecologists. Practice Bulletin No 178: Shoulder dystocia. *Obstet Gynecol.* 2017;129(5):e123–33. doi: 10.1097/AOG.0000000000002043

Royal College of Obstetricians and Gynaecologists. *Shoulder Dystocia.* Green – top Guideline No. 42. 2nd edition, 2012 Mar

Sentilhes L, Sénat MV, Boulogne AI, Deneux-Tharaux C, Fuchs F, Legendre G, Le Ray C, Lopez E, Schmitz T, Lejeune-Saada V. Shoulder dystocia: Guidelines for clinical practice from the French College of Gynecologists and Obstetricians (CNGOF). *Eur J Obstet Gynecol Reprod Biol.* 2016;203:156–61. doi: 10.1016/j.ejogrb.2016.05.047

Cord prolapse

Fischer RL. Umbilical cord prolapse: Are maneuvers always necessary to relieve cord compression? *Am J Obstet Gynecol.* 2022;226(5):746. doi: 10.1016/j.ajog.2021.12.009

NHS Resolution. *Case Story: Good Practice in Managing Umbilical Cord Prolapse.* NHS, 2021 Oct

Wong L, Kwan AHW, Lau SL, Sin WTA, Leung TY. Umbilical cord prolapse: Revisiting its definition and management. *Am J Obstet Gynecol.* 2021;225(4):357–66. doi: 10.1016/j.ajog.2021.06.077

Inverted uterus

Haeri S, Rais S, Monks B. Intrauterine tamponade balloon use in the treatment of uterine inversion. *BMJ Case Rep.* 2015;2015:bcr2014206705. doi: 10.1136/bcr-2014-206705

Johnson NP, Bishop E, Buist R. Hydrostatic replacement of acute inversion of the uterus can cause acute pulmonary oedema by intrauterine fluid intravasation. *J Obstet Gynaecol.* 1999;19:544–5

Ogueh O, Ayida G. Acute uterine inversion: A new technique of hydrostatic replacement. *BJOG.* 1997;104:951–2

Wendel MP, Shnaekel KL, Magann EF. Uterine inversion: A review of a life-threatening obstetrical emergency. *Obstet Gynecol Surv.* 2018;73(7):411–17. doi: 10.1097/OGX.0000000000000580

Amniotic fluid embolism

Fitzpatrick KE, van den Akker T, Bloemenkamp KWM, Deneux-Tharaux C, Kristufkova A, Li Z, Schaap TP, Sullivan EA, Tuffnell D, Knight M. Risk factors, management, and outcomes of amniotic fluid embolism: A multicountry, population-based cohort and nested case-control study. *PLoS Med.* 2019;16(11):e1002962. doi: 10.1371/journal.pmed.1002962

Kaur K, Bhardwaj M, Kumar P, Singhal S, Singh T, Hooda S. Amniotic fluid embolism. *J Anaesthesiol Clin Pharmacol.* 2016;32(2):153–9. doi: 10.4103/0970-9185.173356

Sudden maternal collapse

Soar J, Böttiger BW, Carli P, Couper K, Deakin CD, Djärv T, Lott C, Olasveengen T, Paal P, Pellis T, Perkins GD, Sandroni C, Nolan JP. European Resuscitation Council guidelines 2021: Adult advanced life support. *Resuscitation*. 2021;161:115–51. doi: 10.1016/j.resuscitation.2021.02.010

Soskin PN, Yu J. Resuscitation of the pregnant patient. *Emerg Med Clin North Am*. 2019;37(2):351–63. doi: 10.1016/j.emc.2019.01.011

Anaphylaxis

Cardona V, Ansotegui IJ, Ebisawa M, El-Gamal Y, Fernandez Rivas M, Fineman S, Geller M, Gonzalez-Estrada A, Greenberger PA, Sanchez Borges M, Senna G, Sheikh A, Tanno LK, Thong BY, Turner PJ, Worm M. World Allergy Organization anaphylaxis guidance 2020. *World Allergy Organ J*. 2020;13(10):100472. doi: 10.1016/j.waojou.2020.100472

Muraro A, Worm M, Alviani C, Cardona V, DunnGalvin A, Garvey LH, et al. European Academy of Allergy & Clinical Immunology. Food allergy, anaphylaxis guidelines group. EAACI guidelines: Anaphylaxis (2021 update). *Allergy*. 2022;77(2):357–77. doi: 10.1111/all.15032

Simionescu AA, Danciu BM, Stanescu AMA. Severe anaphylaxis in pregnancy: A systematic review of clinical presentation to determine outcomes. *J Pers Med*. 2021;11(11):1060. doi: 10.3390/jpm11111060

Latex allergy

Adeley J, Rowland A. Managing the risk of latex allergy in healthcare workers and patients. *Clin Risk* 1999;5:129–31

Diaz T, Martinez T, Antepara I, et al. Latex allergy as a risk during delivery. *BJOG*. 1996;103:173–5

Eckhout GV Jr, Ayad S. Anaphylaxis due to airborne exposure to latex in a primigravida. *Anesthesiol*. 2001;4:1034–5

Santos R, Hernandez-Ayup S, Galache P, et al. Severe latex allergy after a vaginal examination during labour: A case report. *Am J Obstet Gynecol*. 1997;177:1543–4

Shingai Y, Nakagawa K, Kato T, et al. Severe allergy in a pregnant woman after vaginal examination with a latex glove. *Gynecol Obstet Invest*. 2002;54:183–4

Mid-trimester termination of pregnancy for fetal abnormality

American College of Obstetricians and Gynecologists. Management of stillbirth. *Obstetric Care Consensus*. 2020 Mar;10

Royal College of Obstetricians and Gynaecologists. *Termination of Pregnancy for Fetal Abnormality in England, Wales and Scotland*. Report of a Working Group. London: RCOG:20

Appendix: Guidance for obtaining consent to treatment

Every adult woman of sound mind has a right to determine what can be done with her own body. She has an absolute right to refuse to consent to treatment for any reason, rational or irrational, or for no reason at all, even where the decision may lead to her own death. A healthcare provider who treats a woman without her consent could be liable in negligence or in the crime of battery. In the context of the following guidance, 'treatment' includes diagnostic procedures.

Good practice requires the provider to ensure that the woman understands what is proposed and consents to it, before proceeding with treatment or investigation. Where some form of consent has been given, it is important not to exceed the consent given or to carry out a procedure unrelated to the consent.

Who gives consent?

No one can legally give consent on behalf of an adult of sound mind. A spouse or other relative may not give consent or withhold consent if the woman is competent.

How valid is a consent?

The following are necessary for a consent to be valid:

- The woman must have the capacity to make the decision.
- The woman must make the decision without undue influence.
- The woman must be given sufficient information about the treatment.

If there is any doubt about the capacity of the woman, then the consultant should be informed. Guidance can be obtained from *Assessment of Mental Capacity: Guidance for Doctors and Lawyers* (see 'Further reading' at the end of this appendix). In some cases, it might be necessary to seek a court declaration.

Consent should not be obtained under duress. Where there is a recognized undue influence, this should be reported to the supervising consultant or senior midwife.

The professional obtaining consent should declare any potential conflict of interest.

The woman should be given sufficient time to consider the information given. For elective procedures, a reasonable interval should elapse between obtaining consent and performing treatment.

For emergency procedures, the emphasis should be on explaining in simple terms what the situation is and what treatment is being proposed, to the extent that the emergency allows a meaningful discussion. It is not good practice to chase a woman to sign a consent form while she is being wheeled into the operating theatre. The form signed in such circumstances carries no legal validity.

How much information should be given?

This is generally a matter of clinical judgement, depending on individual needs and the complexity of treatment; but enough information should be given to ensure that the woman understands:

- The nature of the treatment.
- The benefits of the treatment.
- The consequences of the treatment and of refusal of treatment.
- Any substantial risk of the treatment.

Where there are alternatives, these should be discussed, and reasons should be given for recommending a particular option. Oral information should be supplemented with information leaflets wherever possible. The use of such leaflets should be recorded.

Who should obtain consent?

To ensure that the woman is fully informed, it is important that her consent be obtained by the person who will provide the treatment. However, this task may be delegated to any professional who:

- Is suitably trained and competent.
- Has sufficient knowledge of the proposed treatment.
- Understands the risks involved.
- Has access to an appropriate support person.

The person providing the treatment remains responsible for ensuring that a valid consent has been obtained.

When is a written consent required?

Express (as opposed to implied) consent may be oral or written. An oral consent is as valid as a written consent, but written consent provides documentary evidence that a discussion took place.

Where oral consent has been obtained, it should be documented in the notes. This should be sufficient for most non-invasive procedures.

Written consent should be obtained for any procedure or treatment carrying any substantial risk or substantial side effect.

> ! Shorthand and abbreviations should not be used and alterations to the consent form should be avoided.

Special cases

- A minor under 16 can give consent if she is Fraser (Gillick) competent.
- An official link worker should be used if the patient does not speak English.
- Arrangements must be made for patients with hearing or speech disabilities.

Procedures for which written consent should be obtained

- All procedures performed in theatre under local, regional or general anaesthesia
  In an emergency, verbal consent should be obtained which should be witnessed by another care professional. Record the decision and the reasons for proceeding to the emergency delivery without written consent
- Amniocentesis
- Medical termination of pregnancy

Procedures for which verbal consent should be obtained and documented

- Blood transfusion
- Induction of labour
- Vaginal examination in labour
- Rectal examination
- Vaginal examination by a medical student
- Amniotomy, artificial rupture of fetal membranes (ARM)
- Breech vaginal delivery
- Fetal scalp blood sampling
- Instrumental delivery
- ECV
- Epidural analgesia
- Administration of enema/suppository
- Application of a fetal scalp electrode
- Administration of anti-D immunoglobulin
- Syntometrine (ergometrine with oxytocin) injection
- Episiotomy
- Repair of episiotomy
- Administration of vitamin K injection to a baby

If a woman who is deemed to have capacity to consent refuses assisted delivery or caesarean section, even after full consultation and explanation of the consequences for her and for the fetus, her wishes must be respected.

FURTHER READING

Edozien LC. UK law on consent finally embraces the prudent patient standard. *BMJ*. 2015 May 28;350:h2877. doi: 10.1136/bmj.h2877

General Medical Council. *Decision Making and Consent: Guidance on Professional Standards and Ethics for Doctors*. London: General Medical Council, 2020

Royal College of Obstetrics and Gynaecologists. *Obtaining Valid Consent: Clinical Governance Advice, No. 6*. London: Royal College of Obstetrics and Gynaecologists, 2015

Index

Note: page numbers in **bold** indicate a table. Page numbers in *italics* indicate a figure.

A

abnormal lie
  glossary, xxviii
abnormal lie in labour, 130–131
abnormal presentation
  criteria for paediatric attendance at delivery, 54
abnormalities, congenital
  criteria for paediatric attendance at delivery, 54
activated partial thromboplastin time (APTT), 212
acute venous thromboembolism, 192–198
admission to, and discharge from the delivery suite, 10
adult respiratory distress syndrome (ARDS), 161
advance decision
  document, 231
  glossary, xxviii
adverse outcomes in pregnancy, 11, 58, 178
algorithm
  cervical ripening: multipara, *110*
  cervical ripening: nullipara, *110*
  cervical ripening: prior C-section, *111*
  DVT, suspected, *194*
  newborn life support, *66*
  PE, suspected, *195*
amniotic fluid embolism, 215, 225
  disseminated intravascular coagulopathy and, 225
  sudden maternal collapse, 270
amniotomy, 27
  avoiding, 247
  cord prolapse, excluding 264
  fetal demise, 282
analgesia
  birthing pool, 74
  combined spinal epidural, failed, 94
  complications of epidural, 48
  conduct of labour and, 74
  delayed pushing, 95
  discussing, 136
  Entonox, 74
  epidural, 30, 27, 44–46, 55, 106, 207
  epidural, in labour, 43–50
  immediate versus delayed pushing, 52
  instrumental delivery, consideration of, 96
  low-dose epidural, 45
  management of third stage of labour, 55
  midwife or support person, reducing need for, 28
  narcotic, avoiding, 119
  offering, 135, 140, 150, 155
  opioid, 29, 74, 75
  recommending, 168
  regional, 75, 87, 191

analgesics, 57, 128
  narcotic, 28
anaphylaxis, 266–267
antepartum haemorrhage (APH), 210–213
  assessment, 211
  criteria for paediatric attendance at delivery, 54
  definition of, 210
  delivery, 213
  differential diagnoses, 210
  RCOG classification of APH, 210
  placental abruption, 210
  major APH (significant bleeding, 50–1000 mL but not in shock), 211
  massive APH (estimated loss >1000 mL and/or signs of clinical shock), 211
  minor APH (minimal loss, <50 mL on admission), 211
antibiotics, 25
  conservative management, 117
  cover, 150, 180
  erythromycin, 117
  expectant management, 25
  immediate postpartum care, 57
  oral penicillin, 117
  penicillin, 180
  prelabour rupture of membranes at or near term, 76
  prolonged rupture of fetal membranes, 238
  prophylactic, 87, 88, 120, 143, 180, 237
  sepsis, 239
antiphospholipid antibody, 178, 188, 190
antiphospholipid syndrome (APS), 207, 208
antiplatelet antibodies, 205, 206
antithrombin deficiency, 208
anti-Xa assay
  activity, peak, 44
  inhibitors, 187
  glossary, xxviii
APH, *see* antepartum haemorrhage
apnoea, 49, 61
  primary, 64
  secondary, 64
  terminal, 64
APS, *see* antiphospholipid syndrome
APTT, *see* activated partial thromboplastin time
ARDS, *see* adult respiratory distress syndrome
ARM, *see* artificial rupture of fetal membranes
arterial line
  delivery of woman with known risk of haemorrhage, 227
  glossary, xxviii
  heart disease in labour, 150
  high-dependency care and, 92
  massive APH, 212

obese woman in labour, pre-eclamptic, 142
severe pre-eclampsia, 156
artificial rupture of fetal membranes (ARM), 39, 109, 167
asthma, 173–174
atopy and, 274

B

bariatric surgery, 143
basic life support (BLS), 49, 267, 268, 270
beta-sympathomimetic, 115
Bishop score, 25, 26
glossary, xxviii
biosocial approach to woman in labour, 3
birthing pool, 73–75
blood pressure (BP) 23, 27
care of mother, 57
checking, 34, 46, 47
fetal hypoxia, 64
hypertensive women, 51
maternal, 45, 46, 47
monitoring equipment, 44
normal, 35
second stage of labour, 51, 52
systolic below 90 mmHg, 48
very low, 49
blood transfusion
administering, 228–230
management of woman who declines, 231–233
coagulation disorders 202–204
BLS, *see* basic life support
BP, *see* blood pressure
breech extraction, 128, 129
breech presentation, 127, 135
CS for, 85, 130
face presentation mistaken for, 133
multiple delivery, 127
breech vaginal delivery, 136
criteria for paediatric attendance at delivery, 54

C

caesarean section (CS), 85–89
abnormal lie-in-labour, 130
classification of urgency of, 86
Cochrane Review, 25
delayed elective, 88
elective, 86, 168, 197
emergency, 87
epidurals, 43
epilepsy and, 175
high-risk cases, 88
HIV and preparation for, 251
Maternal Satisfaction for CS (MSCS), 5
meconium-stained fluid at, 63
medication to reduce the risk of aspiration syndrome, 85
planned, 3
postoperative care, 88
preparations, 85
prophylactic antibiotics, 88, 237
surgical procedure, 87
workplace noise, 87

thromboprophylaxis, 89, 187
trial of vaginal delivery after previous CS, 106–107
cardiography, 260
cardiolipin antibody, 190
cardiologist, 180
cardiomyopathy, 92, 152
cardiopulmonary resuscitation (CPR), 259, 272
cardiotocograph (CTG)
classification of, 32, **33**
list of NICE intrapartum care of quality statements, 3
suspicious or pathological, 32
cardiopulmonary resuscitation (CPR), 160
cardiorespiratory arrest, 160
cardiovascular
collapse, 49, 270
disease, hydralazine not to be used in event
of, 158
dysfunction, 115
maternal risk, 149
central venous pressure (CVP)
arterial line and, 212, 227
glossary, xxviii
line, insertion of, 156
monitoring, 163
see also, postpartum haemorrhage: checklist
cerebrospinal fluid (CSF), 45, 48
cerebrovascular
accident, 154, 270, 272
disease, 286
childhood sexual abuse
woman with history of, 71–72
chorioamnionitis, 25
clinical evidence of, 114
HIV and, 249
preterm uterine contractions, 118, 121
PROM and, 199
steroids and, 118
suspected, 37
chorionicity
confirming, 129
glossary, xxviii
cleidotomy, 262
glossary, xxviii
clinical incidents, 11–13
analysis, 12
confidentiality, 13
learning from, 11
reporting, 12
clotting
abnormalities, 232
baseline, 196
disorder, 85, 100
factor, 202
profile, *see* coagulation profile
screen 155, 259
coagulation profile, 44
glossary, xxviii
coagulopathy, 44, 221
disseminated intravascular, 225
communication
with anaesthetists, 7
between care providers, 6–7

instrumental delivery, 96
  parents experiencing fetal loss, 279
  woman who declines blood transfusion, 232
  woman with history of sexual abuse, 71
congenital abnormalities, 277–279
  as clinical incident, 12
  criteria for paediatric attendance at delivery, 54
  epilepsy, 175
  heart block, 178, 179
connective tissue disorders, 180–181
consent
  for caesarean section, 130
  obtaining, 9, 21, 24, 37, 85, 87, 102,
        215, 229
  obtaining, and documenting, 108
  parental, documenting, 60
  for vaginal exam, 140
  verbal, 38, 299
  verbal, documenting of, 45
  written, 299
cord prolapse, 264–265
Coronavirus disease 2019 (COVID-19)
  action plan, 253
  suspected or confirmed, 74
  pregnant woman with, 253
  thromboembolism prophylaxis, 254
  water birth, 254
  woman with, 253–254
corticosteroid therapy
  antenatal, 114–115
COVID-19, see Coronavirus disease 2019
CPR, see cardiopulmonary resuscitation
CRP, see C-reactive protein
C-reactive protein (CRP)
  conservative management, 117
  elevated, 116
CS, see caesarean section
CSF, see cerebrospinal fluid
CTG, see cardiotocograph
CVP, see central venous pressure
cyanosis, 61, 270

D

DDAVP, see desmopressin acetate
D-dimer, 193
  FDP/D-dimer 271
  glossary, xxviii
deceleration
  cardiotocograph, **33**
  as complication, 34
  late, 35–36
  presence or absence of, 32
  second stage of labour, 36
deep venous thrombosis (DVT)
  anticoagulant therapy for 194
  personal or family history of, 188, 190
  previous, 192
  regional analgesia and risk of, 191
  risk assessment for, 85
  suspected, 193
desmopressin acetate (DDAVP), 203, 204

diabetes
  criteria for paediatric attendance at delivery, 54
  diabetes mellitus, 167–171
  gestational, 169
  diabetic ketoacidosis, 172
diamorphine, see opioids
DIC, see disseminated intravascular coagulopathy
diclofenac, 157, 173
disseminated intravascular coagulopathy (DIC), 225
DVT, see deep venous thrombosis
dystocia
  glossary, xxviii
  shoulder, 261–263

E

early warning score (EWS), 14
  chart, 88
  documenting, 156
  grid, 92, **93**
ECG, see electrocardiography
echocardiography, 152, 153
  transesophageal, 271
eclampsia, 164–166
ECV, see external cephalic version
elective caesarean section, see caesarean section
electrocardiography (ECG)
  arrhythmia, women with history of, 150
  continuous, 90, 92
  magnesium sulphate blood levels, 165
  magnesium toxicity, 160
  peripartum cardiomyopathy action plan, 153
  severe pre-eclampsia, 156
emergency caesarean section, see caesarean section
epidural analgesia
  acute venous thrombosis, 198
  bladder care, 57
  BP recording, 27
  bupivacaine, 46
  catheter, blood-stained, 57
  catheter, removal of, 57, 191
  coagulopathy, 44
  complications of, 48
  contractions and administration of, 47
  contraindications for, 43
  delayed pushing, 95
  discontinuation of, 50
  dural tap, 96
  failed intubation, 94
  fetal heart rate and, 35
  first stage of labour, 30
  immediate versus delayed pushing, 52
  indications for, 43
  informing woman of risks and benefits of, 30
  insertion of spinal/epidural block, 191
  intramuscular pethidine and, 45
  in labour, 43–50
  local anaesthetic toxicity and, 49
  mandatory, 145
  offer, 106, 135, 140, 150, 155
  passive phase of labour, 51
  pudendal block in place of, 137

recommend, 130, 174
removal of epidural catheter, 191
second stage of labour, 48
siting, difficulty in, 142
spinal-epidural, combined 45
third stage of labour, 55
vertex, non-visibility of, 51
thrombophilia, 207
epidurals, 43, 56, 142
see also, anaesthetic
epilepsy, 73, 175–177
after delivery, 176
after seizure, 176
indications for caesarean section, 175
management of fits in labour, 175
management in labour, 175
episiotomy, 70
EUA, *see* examination under anaesthetic, 221
examination under anaesthetic (EUA), 221
EWS, *see* early warning score

F

falx cerebri, 12
glossary, xxviii
FBC, *see* full blood count
FBS, *see* fetal blood sampling
FDP, *see* fibrin degradation product
female genital cutting, 140
Female Genital Mutilation Act 2003, 141
fetal abnormality
mid-trimester termination for, 284–286
fetal bleeding disorders, 32
fetal blood sampling (FBS)
<34 weeks, avoiding, 119
buttock, 136
contraindications to, 28, 36, 37, 133
full cervical dilation, 38
scalp, 37, 38, 100
stable, 38
tachycardia, 34
von Willebrand, 203
fetal bradycardia
management of, 34–35
profound unresponsive, 86
prolonged, 37
fetal breathing, 64
fetal demise
intrauterine, 280–283
fetal distress
bradycardia, 259
criteria for paediatric attendance at delivery, 54
fetal heart (FH)
abnormal heart rate, 7, 32, 51
auscultation of, 21, 31
deterioration of, 49
monitoring of heart rate, 47
normal heart rate, 24
recording of, 23, 49
tones, 132
fetal loss at 13–23 weeks
checklist for, 279

fetal monitoring, 31–36
classification of cardiotocograph, 32
electronic, 31
intermittent auscultation, 31
late deceleration, 35–36
management of cardiotocograph, 32
management of fetal bradycardia, 34–35
management of fetal tachycardia, 34
suspicious or abnormal trace, 31
fetal scalp electrode (FSE)
avoiding use of, 203, 206, 247
contraindication, 32
difficulty in applying, 140
Hepatitis B and C, 241
fetal tachycardia, 34, 74
FFP, *see* fresh frozen plasma
FH, *see* fetal heart
fibrin degradation product (FDP), 44, 212, 225
D-dimer, 271
fifths palpable, 23, 27, 103
glossary, xxviii
first stage of labour, 168
breech presentation, 136
diabetes mellitus, 168
management of, 27–30
multiple pregnancy, 130
FISH, *see* fluorescence in situ hybridization
fresh frozen plasma (FFP), 221
fluorescence in situ hybridization (FISH), 282, 284
FSE, *see* fetal scalp electrode
full blood count (FBC)
acute venous thromboembolism, 193
amniotic fluid embolism, 270
asthma, 173
breech vaginal delivery, 136
diabetic ketoacidosis, 172
disseminated intravascular coagulopathy, 225
elective caesarean section, 197
emergency CS, 87
first stage of labour, 168
haemorrhage, known risk of 226
immune thrombocytepnic purpura, 205
intrapartum sepsis, 239, *245*
intrauterine fetal demise, 281
intravenous cannulation, 22
inverted uterus, 268
major placenta praevia, 214
massive APH, 212
major haemoglobinopathy, 199, 200
multiple pregnancy, first stage of labour, 130
paravaginal haematoma, 257
peripartum cardiomyopathy, 153
placental abruption, 211
postpartum, 161
postpartum haemorrhage, 219
pre-eclampsia, 155
preterm prelabour rupture of membranes, 116, 117
preterm uterine contractions, 118
rupture of uterus, 259
sickle cell crisis, 200
sudden maternal collapse, 273
systemic lupus erythematosus, 178

thrombophilia, 207
trial of vaginal delivery, 106
von Willebrand, 203

G

GBS, *see* group B haemolytic streptococci
gemeprost, 283, 285, 286
gestational
    diabetes, 169
    thrombocytopenia, 209
group B haemolytic streptococci (GBS), 238
    intrapartum GBS prophylaxis, 243
    intrapartum GBS prophylaxis not indicated, 243

H

haemolysis, elevated liver enzymes, low platelets (HELLP)
    coagulopathy, 44, 225
    pre-eclampsia, 44, 154, **156**, 205
haemophilia, 202
    FBS contraindicated, 37
    FSE contraindicated, 32
haemoptysis, 192
haemorrhage and haematological disorders, 185–233
    acute venous thromboembolism and pulmonary embolism,
        192–198
    antepartum haemorrhage, 210–213
    blood transfusion, administering, 228–230
    blood transfusion, management of woman who declines,
        231–233
    coagulation disorders, 202–204
    delivery of woman with known risk of, 226
    disseminated intravascular coagulopathy, 225
    gestational thrombocytopenia, 209
    immune thrombocytopenic purpura, 205–206
    major haemoglobinopathy, 199–201
    major placenta previa, 214–215
    placenta accreta spectrum, 216–217
    postpartum haemorrhage, 219–223, *224*
    retained placenta, 218
    rhesus-negative woman, 185–186
    thromboembolism prophylaxis, 187–191
    thrombophilia, 207–208
HDU, *see* high-dependency unit
heart disease in labour, 149–151
HELLP, *see* haemolysis, elevated liver enzymes,
        low platelets
HELPERR Action Plan 262
Hepatitis B and C, 241
    elective CS and, 241
    FBS contraindicated for, 37
herpes
    active, 37
    FBS contraindicated for, 37
    genital, 247, *248*
herpes simplex virus (HSV), 247
high-dependency unit (HDU)
    early transfer to ITU/HDU, 212, 220
    transfer to ICU and, 16, 92
high vaginal swab (HVS), 243
HIV, *see* human immunodeficiency virus

human immunodeficiency virus (HIV), 249–252
    birthing pool excluded for, 73
    elective CS and, 241
    FBS contraindicated for, 37
    FSE contraindicated for, 32
HSV, *see* herpes simplex virus
HVS, *see* high vaginal swab
hypertension, 55
    adverse outcomes in pregnancy associated with, 178
    contraindications to suppression of labour, 121
    heart disease in labour, 149
    peripartum cardiomyopathy risk factor, 152
    preeclampsia, symptom of, 154, 156, 166

I

immune thrombocytopenic purpura (ITP), 202, 205–206
induction of labour (IOL), 108–117
    acute venous thromboembolism, 197
    artificial rupture of fetal membranes, 157
    fetal abnormality, 285
    intrauterine fetal demise, 282
    preterm prelabour rupture of membranes, 117
    prostaglandin, 167
    pulmonary embolism, 197
    Syntocinon, 22. *See also*, Syntocinon
infection, 237–254
    genital herpes, 247
    Hepatitis B and C, 241–242
    HIV, 249–252
    intrapartum antibiotic prophylaxis for group B
            streptococci, 243–246
    intrapartum sepsis, 239, *245*
    prophylactic antibiotics, 237–238
    woman with COVID-19, 253–254
inherited coagulation disorders, 204
instrumental delivery, 95–103
    abandonment, principle of, 102
    avoiding harm, 95
    choice of instrument, 97
    classification of, 96
    conditions to be fulfilled before, 96
    errors in, 103
    forceps delivery, 100
    glossary, xxviii
    indications for, 96
    management of fetal bradycardia, 35
    trial of, 101
    vacuum-assisted delivery, 99–100
intensive therapy unit (ITU)
    maternal transfer to, 11, 16
intrapartum antibiotic prophylaxis for group B streptococci,
        243–246
intrapartum sepsis, 239, *245*
intrauterine fetal demise, 281
intrauterine growth restriction (IUGR)
    compromised fetus, 111
    contraindications to suppression of labour, 121
    cord-blood sampling, 42
    criteria for paediatric attendance at delivery, 54
    ECV, 139
    pre-eclampsia, 154

SLE, 178
  undiagnosed breech in labour, 135
  urgent CS, 86
  use of birthing pool, 73
intravenous cannulation, 22
intravenous unfractionated heparin, 195
intraventricular haemorrhage (IVH), 120
inverted uterus, 268–269
IOL, *see* induction of labour
ischial spines
  active pushing and, 52
  considerations to be fulfilled before instrument
      delivery, 96
  descent of presenting part in relationship to, 27
  fetal blood scalp sampling at full cervical dilation and, 38
  fetal blood scalp sampling and, 37
  glossary, xxviii
  level of presenting part in relationship to, 21
ITP, *see* immune thrombocytopenic purpura
ITU, *see* intensive therapy unit
IUGR, *see* intrauterine growth restriction
IVH, *see* intraventricular haemorrhage

L

labour, abnormal and high-risk, 85–145
  abnormal lie-in labour, 130–131
  antenatal corticosteroid therapy, 114–115
  breech presentation, 135–137
  caesarean section, 85–89
  deliveries at lower margin of viability, 124–125
  external cephalic version, 138–139
  failed intubation drill, 94
  high-dependency care, 92
  induction of labour, 108–117
  instrumental delivery, 95–105
  malpresentation, 133–134
  multiple pregnancy, 130–152
  obese woman in labour, 142–143
  obstetric patients, recovery of, 90
  occipito-posterior position, 132
  perineal tear, 144–145
  preterm prelabour rupture of membranes, 116–117
  preterm uterine contractions, 118–123
  trial of vaginal delivery after caesarean section, 106–107
  woman with genital cutting, 140–141
labour, normal and low-risk, 21–75
  augmentation of, 39–41
  babies born before arrival at hospital, 69
  birthing pool, 73–75
  cord-blood sampling, 42
  criteria for, 23
  criteria for paediatric attendance at delivery, 54
  epidural analgesia in labour, 43–50
  episiotomy, 70
  fetal monitoring, 31–35
  fetal scalp blood sampling, 37–38
  immediate postpartum care, 57–58
  intravenous cannulation, 22
  management of, 23
  management of first stage of, 27–30
  management of second stage of, 51–53
  management of third stage of, 55–56

meconium-stained amniotic fluid, 62–63
  neonatal resuscitation, 64–68
  newborn, care of, 59–61
  prelabour rupture of membranes (37–42 weeks), 24–26
  vaginal exam, 21
  woman with history of child sexual abuse, 71–72
latex allergy, 274–210
LMWH, *see* low-molecular-weight heparin
low-molecular-weight heparin (LMWH), 194
  contraindications, 196
  dalteparin, 44
  high-risk woman on therapeutic LMWH, 197

M

major haemoglobinopathy, 199–201
major placenta praevia, 214–216
  CS for, 7, 214
  induction of labour, 109
malpresentation, 133–134
  glossary, xxviii
massive APH, 212. *See also*, APH
methicillin-resistant *Staphylococcus aureus* (MRSA), 15, 23
meconium aspiration syndrome, 62
meconium-stained ammonic fluid, 62–63
  ARM and, 39, 109
  care of newborn and, 59
  criteria for paediatric attendance at delivery, 54
  fresh, 31
  intravenous cannulation, 22
  use of birthing pool, 73
medical conditions, 149
  asthma, 173–174
  connective tissue disorders, 180–181
  diabetes mellitus, 167–172
  eclampsia, 164–166
  epilepsy, 175–176
  heart disease in labour, 149–176
  peripartum cardiomyopathy, 152–153
  pre-eclampsia, 154–163
  systemic lupus erythematosus, 178–179
misoprostol, 25, 149, 150, 285
  contraindications, 286
MRSA, *see* methicillin-resistant *Staphylococcus aureus*
multiple pregnancy, 130–152
  artificial rupture of fetal membrane, 109
  criteria for paediatric attendance at delivery, 54
  delivery of woman with known risk of haemorrhage, 226
  elective CS, 86
  epidural analgesia, 43
  intravenous cannulation, 22
  first stage of labour, 130
  Syntocinon, 40
  Syntocinon infusion, 112
  third stage of labour, 55
  use of birthing pool, 73

N

naloxone, 63, 67
neonatal
  lupus, 179
  resuscitation, 64–68

seizures, 11
  unit, 8, 15
  unit, transfer to, 171
neonate
  care of, 170
  immune thrombocytopenic purpura, 206
  inherited coagulation disorders, 204
  intrapartum antibiotic prophylaxis for group b
      streptococci, 244
neonatologists, 8
newborns
  reducing risk in, 86
nifedipine, 121
non-steroidal anti-inflammatory drug (NSAID)
  avoiding, 157, 203
  allergies to, 122
  diclofenac, 157, 173
  peripartum haemorrhage, 180
NSAID, see non-steroidal anti-inflammatory drug
NTD, see neural tube defect
neural tube defect (NTD)
  scan diagnosis of, 285

O

obese woman in labour, 142–143
obstetric emergencies, 257
  amniotic fluid embolism, 270
  anaphylaxis, 266–267
  cord prolapse, 264–265
  inverted uterus, 268–269
  latex allergy, 274–311
  paravaginal haematoma and cervical tear, 257–258, 258
  rupture of uterus, 259
  shoulder dystocia, 261–263
  sudden maternal collapse, 272–273
OP, see occipito-posterior
opioids, 29–30
  diamorphine, 29, 175, 285
  pethidine 29, 45, 63, 74, 175, 201, 206
  remifentanil PCA, 30
occipito-posterior (OP) position, 132

P

paravaginal haematoma and cervical tear, 257–258, 258
  PPH possibly concealed in 272
  suspected, 144
partogram, 9, 27, 74, 106
  glossary, xxviii
patient group direction
  glossary, xxviii
  midwife administration of Vitamin K and naloxone,
      per, 67
  oral Vitamin K, 60
  pain relief per, 29
  Syntocinon infusion per, 22, 40
PDS, see polydioxanone sulphate sutures
perineal tear, 144–145
peripartum cardiomyopathy, 152–153
pethidine, see opioids
placenta
  retained, 218

placental abruption, 210–211
  coagulopathy, 44
  as complication of pre-eclampsia, 154
  as contraindication to suppression of labour, 121
  cord-blood sampling, 42
  ECV, 138
  excluding, 33
  maternal collapse from, 7
  three grades of, 210
  urgent CS, 86
  uterine tenderness, 118
  vaginal bleeding, 35
placenta accreta spectrum, 216–217
placenta previa
  major, 214–215
plasma substitute, 212, 220, 233
  glossary, xxviii
polydioxanone sulphate sutures (PDS), 145
polyhydramnios
  criteria for paediatric attendance at delivery, 54
postpartum, 161
postpartum haemorrhage (PPH), 219
  watch for, 157
PPH, see postpartum haemorrhage
pre-eclampsia, 154–163
preterm prelabour rupture of membranes, 116, 117
preterm uterine contractions, 118
primary apnoea 64
prolapsed cord
  criteria for paediatric attendance at delivery, 54
PROM, see prelabour rupture of fetal membranes
prothrombin gene mutation, 207
prothrombin time (PT), 187, 221
  clotting profile compromising, xxviii
PT, see prothrombin time

R

remifentanil PCA, see opioids
respiratory distress (infant)
  baby not in, 62
  indications for instrumental delivery, 96
  reducing risk in newborns, 86
  transfer to neonatal unit in case of, 171
  See also, ARDS
Rhesus (Rh) isoimmunization, 54, 138
  glossary, xxviii
rupture of uterus, 259
  ECV, 138
  excluding, 269

S

SBAR, see situation, background, assessment,
      recommendation
SCBU, see special-care baby unit
secondary apnoea, 64. See also, apnoea
sepsis, 239
sexual abuse, see childhood sexual abuse
sickle cell crisis, 200
situation, background, assessment, recommendation (SBAR),
      14, 16
SLF, see systemic lupus erythematosus

special-care baby unit (SCBU), 61, 63
    admittance to, 245
    alerting, 120
    informing, 124
specialty trainee (ST), 6
spontaneous rupture of fetal membranes (SROM), 251
SROM, *see* spontaneous rupture of fetal membranes
ST, *see* specialty trainee
stillbirth and congenital abnormalities, 279
    checklist for fetal loss at 13–23 weeks, 279
    intrauterine fetal demise, 280–283
    mid-trimester termination for fetal abnormality, 284–286
sudden maternal collapse, 272–273
Syntocinon
    abnormal lie-in labour, 130
    acceleration of labour with, 40
    APH and, 213
    augmentation with, 40, 41, 130
    breech extraction, 128
    breech presentation, 127
    elective caesarean section, 197
    induction of labour, 22, 26, 108–109
    infusion, 25, 31, 33, 35, 40, 41, 53, 87, 105, 112, 117, 161
    low-dose regime of, 112
    occipito-posterior position, 132
    pre-eclampsia, 161, **162**
    postpartum haemorrhage, 219
    retained placenta, 218
    secondary uterine inertia, 136
    uterine hyperstimulation, 113
    third stage of labour, 129
    trial of vaginal delivery after C-section, 107
Syntometrine, 55
    heart disease in labour, do not use, 150
    multiple pregnancy, do not use, 127
    severe pre-eclampsia, do not use, 157
systemic lupus erythematosus (SLF), 178–179
    differential diagnoses of thrombocytopenia in
        pregnancy, 205

T

TED, *see* thromboembolism-deterrent stockings
terminal apnoea, 64
thromboembolism-deterrent stockings (TED), 188, 189, 190,
        191, 197, 198
thromboembolism prophylaxis, 187–191
    woman with COVID-19, 254
thrombophilia, 207
    VTE and, 193
thromboprophylaxis, 89
    caesarean section, 187
    vaginal deliveries 189
tocolysis, 41
    cord prolapse, 265
    glossary, xxviii

major placenta praevia, 214
second stage of labour/Syntocinon, 41
uterine hyperstimulation, 112, 113
tocolytic
    beta-sympathomimetic, 115
    ECV, 139
    glossary, xxviii
    monitoring of women on, 123
    preterm labour, 151
    transfer of woman with fetus in utero, 15
    turtle sign, 262
transfer of care between professionals, 14–16
    early transfer to HDU or ITU, 212, 220
    handover by clinical staff, 14
    transfer back to the community or GP care, 15
    transfer between hospitals with the fetus in utero, 15
    transfer of emergencies from primary care, 14
    transfer of care between consultants, 15
    transfer to ICU and HDU, 16, 92
turtle sign, 262

U

uterus
    inverted, 268
    rupture of uterus, 138, 259, 269

V

vaginal delivery
    breech, 7, 136
    classification of instrumental, 96
    errors in instrumental, 103
    management of, 250
    meconium-stained fluid at, 62
    thromboprophylaxis in, 189
    trial of, after previous caesarean section, 106–107
vaginal bleeding
    uncontrolled, 15
vaginal examination (VE), 21
vaginal swab, 24, 282
VE, *see* vaginal examination
venous thromboembolism (VTE)
    D-dimer diagnostic value, 193
    minimizing risk of, 187
    pyrexia confused with, 239
    thrombophilia testing in presence of, 193
    VTE prophylaxis, 90, 142
    women with previous VTE, 208
Vitamin K, 60
    babies born before arrival at hospital, 69
    midwife administration of, 67
von Willenbrand disease, 202, 203
von Willebrand Factor (vWF), 203, 204
VTE, *see* venous thromboembolism
vWF, *see* von Willebrand Factor

Printed in the United States
by Baker & Taylor Publisher Services